Introduction to Dr

Introduction to Dramatherapy provides a theoretical framework for the practice of dramatherapy, and examines the relationship between the 'self' and the 'other'; the understanding of which, the author argues, is key to harnessing the full potential of dramatherapy as a healing medium.

In three sections: 'The Theatre and the World', 'Foundations of Dramatherapy' and 'Dramatherapy and its Applications', both the theory and practice of dramatherapy are explored. In Part I, the individual is introduced in terms of the dramatic metaphor, concentrating on the central issue of identity and the mediation between the internal and external worlds. In Part II the elements that make up dramatic reality, specifically play narrative and role, are examined, and in the final part we witness the value of dramatherapy in practice in a range of clinical settings.

This is not simply a 'how to do dramatherapy' book – it provides an essential foundation in the theory of the subject that will be of great interest to those studying or practising dramatherapy.

Salvo Pitruzzella is a dramatherapist, psychodramatist and theatre teacher. He works both in private practice and as a chartered dramatherapist in a care and rehabilitation centre for teenagers with personality disorders. He is founder and director of the first dramatherapy training course in Italy.

Introduction to Dramatherapy

Person and threshold

Salvo Pitruzzella

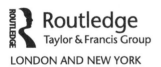

Routledge
Taylor & Francis Group

LONDON AND NEW YORK

First published 2004
by Brunner-Routledge
Published 2016 by Routledge
2 Park Square, Milton Park, Abingdon, Oxon, OX14 4RN

Simultaneously published in the USA and Canada
by Routledge
711 Third Avenue, New York, NY 10017

Brunner-Routledge is an imprint of the Taylor & Francis Group

Copyright © 2004 Salvatore Pitruzzella

Typeset in Times by
Keystroke, Jacaranda Lodge, Wolverhampton
Paperback cover design by Sandra Heath

British Library Cataloguing in Publication Data
A catalogue record for this book is available from the British Library

Library of Congress Cataloging-in-Publication Data
Pitruzzella, Salvo.
  Introduction to dramatherapy : person and threshold / Salvo
Pitruzzella ; foreword by Roger Grainger, afterword by Sue Emmy
Jennings.
    p. ; cm.
  Includes bibliographical references and index.
  ISBN 1-58391-974-0 (hbk.) – ISBN 1-58391-975-9 (pbk.)
  1. Psychodrama. 2. Drama–Therapeutic use.
  [DNLM: 1. Psychodrama–methods. 2. Psychological Theory. WM
430.5.P8 P686i 2004] I. Title.

  RC489.P7P587 2004
  616.89'1523–dc22

                                                    2003019903

ISBN 1-58391-974-0 (hbk)
ISBN 1-58391-975-9 (pbk)

In memory of D.
Theatre did not save his life.

Contents

Acknowledgements

I wish to thank first of all the two people who most encouraged and supported me in the project of this book: Roger Grainger and Sue Emmy Jennings. I had the chance to appreciate not only their deep knowledge of Dramatherapy, but also their truthful caring quality.

The book is the fruit of a 12-year experience in studying and experimenting with drama in therapeutic and educational fields. It shows the marks of countless people I have met: students, clients and colleagues. I have learned something from each of them.

I want to thank Claudio Bonanomi and the staff of the Arts Therapies Training Centre (Lecco, Italy) and the Cooperative 'Il Canto di Los' (Palermo, Italy): they both supported my research and made possible the making of the book.

I thank my wife, Melania, for her joyous bearing my many sleepless nights, and my children, Martino, Ariele and Viola, who have been a constant source of inspiration.

My gratitude is also for friends and colleagues with whom I had discussed the issues of the book: Franco La Cecla, Fabrizio Fiaschini, Aldo Costa, Antonietta Minì, Claudio Bernardi, Robert J. Landy and Peter Slade.

Author's royalties of this book are being assigned to Sue Jennings's social projects in Zarnesti (Romania), which include: Project Wolf for disaffected young people; Avalon Groups for women – including victims of domestic violence; Creative Journeys for people with disabilities.

The Little Girl Named I from *Fairy Tales* © 1950, 1965 by Marion Morehouse Cummings and renewed 1978 by the E.E. Cummings Trust, reprinted by permission of Harcourt, Inc. *The World Saved by Kids* © 1968, Elsa Morante Estate. All rights reserved handled by Agenzia Letteraria Internazionale, Milan, Italy. Every effort has been made to trace

the copyright holders and obtain permission to reproduce Bertolt Brecht's
Description of the Way of Acting of H.W.; Rabindranath Tagore's *Sissu*,
and Robinson Jeffers's *Summer Holiday*. Any omissions brought to our
attention will be remedied in future editions.

Foreword

Entering with my body inside the narration, I participate in it, making it, in its mimetic resonances, a community event. . . . In this sense, the narrative dimension reaffirms the principle of the freedom and the power that we exert over our destiny as human beings able to think and to imagine.

I have chosen this passage from Salvo Pitruzzella's book for two reasons. First, it penetrates to the living, healing hearth of drama and shows it to be therapeutic in the deepest, most human, sense of all. Second, it reveals the most outstanding quality this book possesses – its intense and unashamed humanness. Pitruzzella's writing is rooted in the experiential, emerging all the time from the realities he is describing. He is a *drama*therapist, and his business is with the embodied and not simply with argument and disembodied imagination: 'Entering with my body . . .'. Thus, for him, body is both revealer and thing revealed, 'primal experience and mask . . . the point of departure for a shared dramatic language'.

The author's passion for the things he describes does not involve any blurring of his intellectual grasp, however, concerned as he is with therapy as art, able to overcome the all too familiar distinction between affect and cognition by moving and convincing us at the same time. (This is dramatically illustrated in a powerfully stated exposition of the dynamics of playing, a sphere of human activity in which imagination and actuality, freedom and structure, mingle creatively.)

All in all, this is a resonant piece of writing, particularly in its exploration of the ways in which human personality is conceptualized as mad or sane according to a culture-bound identification of 'mental illness' with specific kinds of loss of interpersonal communication. Through the dramatic processes, those whom Peter Brook has called 'sealed-off souls' may find 'a metaphoric possibility to be revealed in the shape of images that become common heritage, breaking the chains of isolation and showing themselves as places of encounter'.

At the hearth of *Person and Threshold* is the conviction that Dramatherapy is fundamentally experiential rather than technical; or rather that the experience of drawing close to the dynamisms on which personality depends – interactions that are both obvious and hidden – precedes any techniques we may devise in order to regulate and control it. Thus the marriage of personal insight and reflective analysis celebrated by Bruce Wilshire is here consummated in terms of an actual treatment modality. Newcomers to Dramatherapy, and those for whom this is the first experience they have had of any of the arts therapies, will be fascinated by how much it has to contribute to our understanding of what we are accustomed to calling 'ordinary life'. Dramatherapists will find this book personally enriching, as well as professionally stimulating. It is not addressed only to practitioners, however, but to everyone involved in the human search for ways of deepening our awareness of the crucial nature of the relationship between self and other.

Dramatherapy is essentially a liminal experience. It is a special place and time happening *between*, serving as the threshold of a more personal future – an experience of renewal to be recognized and remembered. For me, my own visit to Palermo in the winter of 2001 was such a threshold. This was my first time in Italy. I had been invited over to meet and confer with arts therapists from all over the country. I was surprised and delighted by the warmth and enthusiasm of my welcome. (I realize, now that I know Salvo better, that I had no reason to be surprised!) Never before, since becoming a dramatherapist many years earlier, had I felt so enthusiastic about what I was involved in. Never before had I been so very conscious of the scope and richness, the deep humanity, of Dramatherapy. I am particularly glad to be able to record the fact here, because *Person and Threshold* is the profoundest book about Dramatherapy that I have read.

Roger Grainger

Introduction
A healing theatre

> The arts have to be taken into serious consideration as forms of discovery, of creation, of knowledge amplification, and therefore the philosophy of art should be conceived as an integral part of metaphysics and epistemology.
>
> (Nelson Goodman 1968: 120–1)

The new paradigm

In his seminal book *Role-playing an Identity*, in which the connections are explored between the theatrical metaphor used to describe human reality, and the essence of theatre itself as a mirror of the processes involved in the creation of individual and social identity, the American philosopher Bruce Wilshire hopes for a new renaissance of dramatic art as 'the rite of authorization and authentication that theatre suggests but does not provide: a ceremony in which people gather together at regular intervals in world-time and confirm each other as individuals through progressively articulating their mimetic fusions with others' (Wilshire 1982: 295).

This suggestion implies that drama has the potential to improve the lives of people who meet it. Dramatherapy is a form of dramatic art aimed at enhancing the well-being of the persons involved via the guided exploration on stage of various ways of being in the world and having relationships with other people. The principles that allow such an exploration to take place lie first and foremost in the structure of drama itself.

In order to analyse these principles, we must begin our investigation with the ways in which theatre has attempted to maintain what Wilshire refers to as its implicit promise: to re-establish itself as a ritual of encounter. Therefore, before introducing the contents of this book, I would like to look at some trends in twentieth-century theatre, without which Dramatherapy would never have been born.

Antonin Artaud stands at the root of some of these trends. Artaud (1896–1948) was a writer, dramatist, actor and director, traveller, poet and visionary. He died in solitude after a long stay in a psychiatric hospital. If according to Hillman (1996), one were to attempt to ascribe a *daimon*, an archetypical figure presiding over human destiny, to his extraordinary and restless existence, it would undoubtedly be the figure of Prometheus. Artaud's vision struggles against the chains of everyday perception and shows us 'portions of eternity too vast for the human eye to behold'.[1] Artaud's strong protests against the richly dressed hypocrisy of theatre in his time are the revolt of a frantic soul against 'this distilled boredom in which our soul has been soaking for seven eternities, this infernal grip in which consciences grow mouldy, needing music, poetry and theatre to explode from time to time, but such a small amount that it is not worth mentioning' (*Lettres de Rodez*). However, at the same time his dissent allows theatre to regenerate itself from the ashes, ceasing to be a mere form of bourgeois entertainment, to be enjoyed while seated comfortably in a velvet stall, shedding a tear for the protagonist's fate, and going home after the performance, satisfied, consoled and well fed.

According to Artaud theatre can – and *must* – be something else. First of all, it must be a supreme creative act: drama does not replicate the world mimetically, but creates it. It is not a copy but a *double*: 'not of that everyday direct reality, of which it has become an inert copy, idle and sweetened, but of another reality, risky and typical, where principles, as dolphins, once glimpsed, hurriedly vanish in deep waters' (Artaud 1964: 165). Theatre unveils, but it is an unveiling that can be fatal, as the vision of the naked goddess for the hunter Atheon. Artaud's catharsis is not just a purge, but death and rebirth. And theatre unveils as the plague does: infection, the extreme limits to which human existence is pushed, and dissolution are the requirements for regeneration, springing from the actor's sacrifice on stage. Certainly, because according to Artaud the protagonist of the death/rebirth cycle, more than the audience, is the actor; he has to prepare himself for the sacrifice through special discipline. As we see, Artaud demolishes the pillars of Aristotle's theatrical aesthetics, which have supported the theatrical edifice for many centuries, implicitly or explicitly, thus suggesting a return to its origins: to primeval rites and shamanism.

It was inevitable that all post-war theatre take up Artaud's challenge, especially from the sixties on, in a time when a multitude of signs from all spheres of life pointed to a palingenetic transformation. 'The times they are a-changing,' sang Bob Dylan, combining a biblical millenarism with his message of protest. And the philosopher Herbert Marcuse invoked 'the liberation of sensibility and human feelings, not as a private fact, but as a force to be employed for the transformation of people's life and environment' (in Cooper 1968: 185).

Radical changes were flooding the theatre. First of all, it was released from the confines of academies and professional companies and spread into the society, creating an overall picture of widespread theatricality. Spontaneous groups were born, researching and experimenting; basements, warehouses and streets were rediscovered as stages; theatre became within everybody's reach, and everyone had the chance to participate in a creative dramatic experience through workshops. The transformation of the rehearsal room into a workshop is not a mere technical fact but a structural change that implicates an epistemological shift in the very conception of the dramatic process. Unlike what happens in the traditional theatre, where the actors' work, intentionally finalized to the performance, is planned according to a precise project of the director (and often of the production), the workshop is a place of collective research, in which the theatre is generated by the creative process itself, often assuming the form of a quest for knowledge. Dramaturgy becomes a work in progress that can integrate upsetting elements in an ever-changing context, rather than eliminating them as 'noise' – as happens in dully intentional processes.

It is impossible to provide an exhaustive account about poetics and the formal result of the many trends that, enlightened by Artaud, turned theatre customs upside down.[2] I shall simply try to list a few common traits pertaining to the change of paradigm mentioned above, whose aim is to root theatre once more in the community as a place of encounter and transformation.

The most important change involves the shifting of borders between theatre and life: first and foremost the one between mimesis and creation. What happens on stage is not a mere representation (or re-presentation) of something resembling the world off stage, but a collective ritual in which the audience is included in a unique and unrepeatable event, at the end of which everybody, actors and audience alike, is changed as a result.[3] Actors are the officiants of this rite, so they must undergo special training. It is not just a matter of learning to move and talk in a certain way or to show emotions. What they are asked to do is to search for the innermost sources of individual expression.

This shifting of borders between what Wilshire distinguishes as the world and the 'world' (the former being the area of everyday reality as it is usually shared by most people; within it the 'world' of drama is placed at a qualitatively different level of reality, as we will see later) is mirrored in the physical conditions that are required for the theatre event to happen.

In its recovered ritual essence, theatre regards scenery as unnecessary, reducing it to a bare minimum. As such, there are no more illusionary sets: the flesh, blood and breath of the actors are enough for the rite to be celebrated. The stage itself takes on new dimensions. The separation between actors and audience is blurred and a global event space is proposed, something nearer to the *temenos* (sacred enclosure) than to the *theatron*.

Everything aims at essentiality. 'I can take an empty space and call it bare scene. A person crosses this empty space while somebody else looks at him, and this is what is necessary for a theatrical action to be undertaken,' wrote Peter Brook (1968: 1). This implies that any place can become a stage by virtue of an agreement between people, as theatre, in its most authentic essence, as Jerzy Grotowski maintained 'is what happens between the actor and the spectator'.

Another theatrical trend to which Dramatherapy is greatly indebted is Improvisation (Impro).[4] It was also born around the sixties as a reaction to what Brook (1968) called 'deadly theatre'. It models itself not on the rite but on another ancient collective activity as old as humankind itself: the game. Like musical improvisation, theatrical improvisation aims at the group creation of a spontaneous and unpredictable artistic event, founded on simple rules of interaction and composition and, above all, on synchrony among people. The actor's preparation is also of utmost importance. Improvisers must know how to improvise. Therefore they must develop qualities of inventiveness, spontaneity and imagination that allow them to embody the stories resulting from the collective interactions on stage; as well as qualities of attention, intuition and empathy that allow them to join productively the group's creative process. They must know how to risk venturing into an action without knowing how it will end, and to risk making mistakes from which they must somehow recover.

In the training process, the actor learns how to move inside a theatrical grammar that is mainly a relational one. Its rules are: to accept offers; to pay attention to and support others; and to make the action advance. This work requires a firm insight into human relationships, which allows the actor to sense the rhythms of others' actions and to tune himself with them in an open, natural way.

The Improvisation performance lives in the relational moment between actors and audience. What the spectator sees is not the more or less successful representation of a story but the creative challenge of the actor with himself.

Psychodrama deserves separate treatment, a discipline akin to Dramatherapy to the extent that at times they appear very similar or even identical. We will see later how a few technical differences between Dramatherapy and Psychodrama procedure, as the latter is currently applied, are hinting at many meaningful differences in the theoretical models.

The fact remains that some important intuitions of Moreno regarding the theatre-life connections are essential facets of the conceptual paradigm of Dramatherapy. Jacob Levi Moreno (1889–1974) was gifted with multiform and rebellious talent. He studied medicine in the Vienna of Freud, but he practised as a physician for only a few years, turning his interests instead to education, social problems and theatre. In particular, he founded the Steigreiftheatre (Spontaneity Theatre), an experimental improvisational theatre. This experience was a privileged observatory of human relations for Moreno, and it allowed him to begin building his model of therapeutic theatre, focused on the dramatic concepts of *role* and *catharsis* and on the philosophical–psychological concepts of *tele* and *spontaneity/creativity*.

The structure of Psychodrama is ingeniously simple. The theatrical script is replaced by the account of events in people's lives that involve some problematic personal issues. The protagonist, helped by the Psychodrama director and by the group, explores the emotional resonances, the motivations and the meanings of them, and he experiments on stage with other possible points of view and alternative developments of the enacted stories.

Starting from these theatrical premises, Moreno founded the first real group psychotherapy. Psychodrama is actually known and practised today as group psychotherapy, with definite emphasis placed on the distance from its theatrical origins. In many of its current applications Psychodrama as group psychotherapy has felt the need to free itself from Moreno's theoretical models (models that, given the exuberant and restless personality of the founder, can seem at times obscure or confused) to link to other psychotherapies, mainly in the psychoanalytic area. This shift has granted Psychodrama citizenship in the psychological establishment, but it has strongly limited its possibilities, by tying it to settings and fields of application specific to traditional psychotherapies.

Three hypotheses for a healing theatre

From these astonishing metamorphoses of dramatic art, that gives up the trappings of illusion and appears essentially as a meeting of people, some hypotheses spring forth on the nature of theatre itself and on the primary processes that constitute it. These hypotheses form the humus from which the practice of Dramatherapy has developed in the last 30 or so years[5] and continues to bear fruit:

1   The actor as an agent of change.
2   Drama as the essence of theatre.
3   Theatre as metaphor.

The actor as an agent of change

In his attempt to formulate the meaning of tragedy in philosophical terms,[6] Aristotle brings the medical concept of *catharsis* into an aesthetical context, underlining the regenerative effect that the performance has on the spectator. Aristotle doesn't say very much about the actor. It seems that he can be reduced to a mere technical tool for the exposure of a poetic text: a mere instrument, just like a brush or a chisel. The skill required of the actor[7] is just to simulate, to lend body and voice to the features and thoughts of somebody else. This image of the actor as a pseudo-technician has subtly permeated the entire history of the theatre, as we will see later in detail. Actually, from the point of view of the actor as a person, it is only a cover for (or at times a defence against) internal shake-ups that happen throughout the whole dramatic process. Anyone who has ever personally experienced a theatrical journey, even if only in a workshop or at school, can testify that the experience leaves deep marks, at times indelible, on the soul. These are marks that can sometimes be very negative: I have personally witnessed states of psychic uneasiness (latent psychosis?) revealed by particularly intense theatrical experiences. What is more, I have seen so many people benefit from the theatrical experience in terms of personal health, improving their self-confidence, self-awareness, sense of irony and open-mindedness.

Dramatherapy tries to direct this transformative energy produced in drama toward the improvement of the participants' lives. Naturally, we are only stating a principle here, but it is important to note that in the origins and development of Dramatherapy this principle does not derive only from the implicit or explicit theories of the new theatrical paradigm. On the contrary, it is always rooted on experience: all the Dramatherapy pioneers have had a firsthand theatrical experience in their personal background. I can personally add that the majority of my students start the training already convinced that theatre can transform life, a conviction based on personal experience. We can furthermore affirm that it is a heuristic principle based on evidence. Putting this principle into effect means not limiting ourselves to a generic statement like 'drama does us good'. We must instead ask ourselves the question 'why does drama do us good?', while avoiding the tautological answer 'drama does us good because it is theatre', and taking into consideration the issue of the responsibility of proposing drama to others as a means for healing. Dramatherapy tries to scan the dramatic process deeply in order to understand how it works. To do this, it resorts not only to artistic tools that have to do with intuition, poetic imagination, and aesthetics feeling, but also to scientific tools that have to do with thought, deduction and empirical research. The comparison with philosophical, psychological, sociological and anthropological models is inevitable, as we will see in greater detail later.

Drama as the essence of the theatre

What are the necessary conditions that allow these intrinsic, transformative factors to emerge in theatre? Let's turn the question around by putting it into the following terms: which elements among those that we traditionally associate with the theatre can be removed without cancelling its transformative potentiality? First, the whole theatrical technical apparatus (the illusion machine): the stage, scenery, costumes, and props. What is needed is a physical space that can be redefined as a threshold place.

The script also becomes unnecessary. Dramatic action must certainly tell a story. Unlike dance, which can be pure, abstract movement, the theatre cannot live without the narrative dimension of the 'fabula', of the soul's tale. But the dramatic action cannot need a pre-existing script: on the contrary, the script can spring from it, or better from the creative process sustaining it. In this sense, the whole dramaturgy of the new theatrical paradigm can be defined as dynamic dramaturgy.

A physical place and a story to be told: this is what is needed for the dramatic event to take place. And the dramatic event is the epiphany of a story, or many stories, from the 'there and then' to the 'here and now'. This requires that dramatic time be special: it interrupts the rhythmic flow of everyday time and accepts particular rules that apply to the dramatic space as well. In this special space/time dimension actions are enacted and stories are told, stories that deal with human life as a whole: values, thoughts, feelings, emotions and desires that belong to the soul of the individual in its relationship with other souls. Most important of all, even the actor's technique becomes unnecessary. To perform those actions, actors don't have to be 'make-believe technicians'; they are only people living an experience. The limits to their expressive skills – serious as they can be, as in the case of disabled people – are not obstacles, but become elements of a shared language.

The theatre of Dramatherapy can be reduced to these primary structures: space/time, story/action, actor/spectator. The terms of this last couplet can be interchangeable, or even be inner features of the same individual. In a play one can both act and observe others' and even one's own actions. In order to do this one must be able to see oneself through the eyes of others, and allow others to do the same.

Theatre as metaphor

A first approach to the art of theatre can be made by considering its dramatic essence: a meeting among people in a place that is different from the everyday space/time, in which someone tells a story through actions and somebody else observes. In this sense, theatre is a universal form and is universally comprehensible. It could be said that we all have the potential to immediately recognize that an action is drama through simple signs. This potential has its roots deep within us, and it is dominant in children's play. Dramatherapy defines it as 'the *as if* principle'. If therefore a dramatic intelligence is deeply rooted in human beings, it means that drama has many things to tell us about human nature.

The theoretical research of Dramatherapy has turned towards this hypothesis at two different levels:

1   The analogy between the primary structures of drama and the processes that govern the development of the relational personality, both in interpersonal and intrapersonal terms. In writing about the dramatic point of view, Robert Landy states: 'In daily life, as in the theatre, the people or the actors assume *Personae* or they play roles to express the sense of their own identity and desires' (1995: 7). Reflections on how these roles are generated, developed and dynamically articulated in the interaction with others, and how they are entwined and animated within us, describe a model of identity and relationships that can help us to understand the nature of both individual and social uneasiness.

2   The aesthetic features in which drama is manifested – that is to say
    the actor/role tension, the patterns in which roles and events are
    interwoven on stage and the rhythms of the dramatic interaction –
    can be seen as signs by which the internal world of the actor reveals
    itself in his relationship with others inside a particular framework
    defined by *as if*. These features may tell us therefore about people's
    inner lives. Acknowledging them may help people to recognize
    the 'various circumstances and factors that limit and distort the
    relationships that we have with others and with ourselves, and to
    reduce their power on us' (Grainger and Andersen-Warren 2000).
    Given these premises, the fact that Dramatherapy dramaturgy is
    dynamic – not rigid or tied to a text, but on the contrary in constant
    transformation – is very significant. It confirms the principle that life
    is not necessarily subjected to a fixed script, written by others, by
    external circumstances or by human weakness. We can write the text
    of our life, and modify it according to our desires and needs,
    negotiating this transformation with others in terms of respect and
    cooperation.

To conclude this brief overview of the theatrical roots of Dramatherapy, which also serves to provide an historical and cultural context,
we can summarize Dramatherapy's theatrical foundations as follows:

- the principle of *effectiveness*, which implies that the dramatic process
  changes the people involved;
- the principle of *essentiality*, which implies the opportunity for anyone
  to participate in the process, regardless of their acting or general
  expressive abilities;
- the principle of *meaning*, which implies the possibility to understand
  the process and to use it for specific objectives.

How these principles have developed to become part of a method will be
the subject of the chapters that follow.

The journey

We will now examine the structure of this book in greater detail. Part I,
'The Theatre and the World' deals with the formation and articulation
of the human person in its relational sphere in terms of the dramatic
metaphor. Our discussion begins with the theme of identity and its
disguises with reference to Wilshire's philosophy of drama, as well as to

the concept of Persona in Carl Gustav Jung and the socio-theatrical theories of Erving Goffmann, and continues with the problem of individual authenticity in the world of relationships. Drama emerges at this point as a place of possible mediation between the external and internal world, and reflections on the tension between actor and character serve as an introduction to the concept of *dramatic reality*, a concept that is at the heart of the theoretical model of Dramatherapy. 'Dramatic reality,' writes Roger Grainger (1997: 2), 'is a special and secure form of reality in which one is allowed to experiment.'

Part II, 'Foundations of Dramatherapy', examines the elements that make up this particular form of reality: play, narrative and role. Each of these elements includes some healing factors, which we will try to highlight. Chapter 4, entitled 'Structures', looks at the conditions which are necessary in order that drama maximize its healing potential. Emphasis is placed on the group and the positive changes that it is able to produce, the dramatic process and its articulation, and finally the therapist's roles, competences and limits.

Part III, 'Dramatherapy and its Applications', focuses on some of Dramatherapy's application fields (mental health, addictions and disabilities). We do not claim to exhaust the complexity of the related issues, but we will simply try to outline a *dramatic point of view* upon them, reflecting on the processes that Dramatherapy can set off.

Part I

The theatre and the world

Remember that here you are nothing but an actor of a play, which will be brief or long according to the desires of the poet. And if he wants you to represent the character of a beggar, study to represent it properly. The same is true if the character assigned to you is that of a lame man, of a judge or of a common man. What is wanted from you is only to act well, whatever character is destined to you: to choose belongs to another.

(Epictetus)

The theatre and the world

Chapter 1

Person

PERSON AND MASK

> You are right to doubt everything, to say the very least . . . I remember
> myself as a little boy, when my father would come to bid me good night.
> Flickering and sputtering all the while, the candle would light up his
> face and it alone, and atrocious doubts would assail me: was that man
> really my father or was he perhaps an impostor? Was he even a man?
> And so on . . . In the end I would bid him good night with a sort of
> complicity, pretending not to notice, not wanting to make a fool
> of myself in front of him or to give in to my fears. . . . But what the devil
> am I saying! I've gone as far as to recount childhood memories!
>
> (Tommaso Landolfi 1958)

The word 'person'

Words sometimes tell stories. The fortune of the word *person* has
fascinated me for a long time. Used in many European languages to define
the complete and complex totality of the single human being, it was
formerly used, as is well known, to mean *mask*. Is this a reversal of
meaning? Is it possible that the term used to denote an object, which helps
to change one's identity by concealing the previous identity (that of the
actor) and assuming a new one (that of the character), succeeds in
expressing the concept of the oneness and permanence of the individual?
Or might it be useful to reflect upon possible shifts and intersections of
the two semantic fields?

It is certain that during the Middle Ages the Latinate languages had to
coin a new word to define the artificial face used in theatre or at carnivals
(no longer in sacred places but in secular ones). There are no certain
hypotheses to explain the origins of the word *mask*. In the folklore of

northern Italy *maschera* or *masca* means the witch, an ancient and demonic creature.

In time, the term person came to be used to designate physical presence and appearance (we must not forget that the Greek equivalent *prosopon* also had the meaning of visage, or face).

Person draws the visible and recognizable outlines of the individual, and it implies being seen. We could even maintain that it is somehow the act of being recognized by another that bestows identity on the person. In Mozart/Da Ponte's *Don Giovanni*, the protagonist slips into the rooms of Donna Anna in disguise. He is able to seduce her because she mistakes him for her fiancé, Don Ottavio. But Don Giovanni is not dressed to resemble Don Ottavio, nor does he give signs that can lead her to recognize him as such. It is Donna Anna's process of discernment that allows the identification to take place.

Let's try to reconstruct the scene: at first, she sees a figure. She must decide whether it is a shadow, a vision, or even a ghost. No, it is a person. At this point the second phase of the identification process begins, based on the characteristics of the context. Who can enter my room at this time? Donna Anna proceeds by elimination: it cannot be my servant, who would never enter my room without knocking, nor my father, who is not back yet, I know for sure. Who can it be then? The best solution is that he is my fiancé and future husband. In making this decision, Donna Anna completes the recognition process, even succeeding in identifying her beloved in the physical form of the person standing next to her. That generic person has become a particular Person with a name and a story.

Name and story, together with physical appearance, are elements that allow us to distinguish one person from another. In this sense we can consider the concept of person as a marker of the temporal continuity of identity. 'Mario Rossi, son of Giuseppe and Maria Bianchi, born in Rome on 1 January 1980 married to Maria Verdi, etc.' Name and story. In extreme cases, a photograph (a testimony of the form). But the name can be changed, and the story can be told in a thousand different ways. Our new neighbour, so polite and kind, can turn out to be a dangerous terrorist on the point of committing an attack. The same persons can be different people in different times and places. Even in absence of a deliberate deception, the same person can otherwise be perceived as different in different environments. A teenager, for instance, can be gloomy and touchy in his own family, and happy and easy with friends. Nevertheless, we wouldn't hesitate to affirm that he is the same person. We start doubting when his actions are so radically different from a range of expectations (the width of the range depends only on us) that we state that he is not himself anymore. We may discover that our child is taking drugs; it is similar to the amazement of Ser Bernardone when his son, Francis of Assisi, appears naked before him. It is not the same person anymore.

So we can figure out Donna Anna's shock when she realizes that the person standing before her is not whom she thought it was. How could this unveiling happen? We can try to imagine the signs through which, in the woman's perception, a process of revision is established. What until now was a particular Person, with all the relational characteristics associated with him (affection, trust, etc.) returns suddenly to the rank (much more disturbing) of generic person. A smell, perhaps? Certainly something inherent to the physical body, and probably to the physical body in action. Not therefore the face, nor the attire (the scene[1] takes place in a dimly lit place), but more likely the feelings provoked by physical contact (which, we can imagine, in the case of Don Giovanni is particularly upsetting), by the rhythm of gestures, by the distance placed between one person and another.

We have a person in front of us, undoubtedly, but the attributes we customarily use to recognize and therefore differentiate someone – name and story – are not available. What remains is a physical body, which enters our perceptive sphere and influences it, forcing us to activate cognitive and emotional processes that allow us to put it into a category, thoughtfully accepted or implicit:

> That persons have material bodies is a necessary truth [. . .]. We cannot identify them without identifying material bodies, and what we must always use to identify, we have to regard as pertaining to the person's identity.
>
> (Wilshire 1982: 149)

Person and body

There is an epistemological radicalism in Wilshire's focus on the body as primary foundation of the person, putting aside at first the theme of the 'I', of self-awareness. The school of thought established by the Cartesian *Cogito* (I think, or I doubt) on the one hand defines man as the reference of man to himself in terms of reflection and conscience, opening the possibility of an ethics of individual responsibility; on the other hand it has introduced the ruinous mind/body dichotomy that has left its mark on Western thought, producing aberrations such as the exaltation of one of the two terms to the total detriment of the other. The derived metaphor of the body as a machine, with or without a 'ghost' in the driver's seat, implies however a drastic idea of separation that experience refuses to accept:

> As Merlau-Ponty, William James, and others have seen, we do not first recognize things and then we manipulate them, but, on a level of recognition that is discovery, manipulate and then recognize. It follows that the body is not first known and then set in motion in the world in terms of the already understood responses and skills of the body, but that the world is understandable only within the context of the already occurring, nonthematic, concernful manipulation and perception of the world, which world includes, as one *eventual* object of studies, the manipulative and perceptive body.
>
> (Wilshire 1982: 155)

At birth, the body of the child is both a physical object and a relational entity. It is provided with an external covering that separates it from the rest of the world and defines it, but to exist (in this case the concept of existence is dynamically interwoven with that of becoming), its covering needs to be permeable. The child needs constant interaction with the world, in terms of nourishment, of contact and of sharing feelings, thereby starting that process of discovery in which knowledge and manipulation are the terms of a unique event:

> I must experience myself as a body identifiable from the others, so my identity must include how I experience others identifying and experiencing my body. Since in the normal course of events there is similarity of response to human bodies by human bodies, I must experience myself to be – and I must be – essentially similar to others.
>
> (Wilshire 1982: 149)

It is also of course a process of differentiation, in the sense that to survive I need to reach a point in which I am able to say 'I', to attribute intentions, desires, feelings and projects to myself, perceiving myself as a figure standing out against the background of the world. Otherwise we risk resembling Italo Calvino's character who becomes a duck, a frog, a fish, then a pear. 'Does he believe he is a duck? – He believes to be the ducks themselves . . . You know Gurdulù: he doesn't pay attention' (Calvino 1960). Gurdulù's lack of attention is the loss of that distance that allows us to enter into a relationship with other things, first and foremost with other human beings, without being mimetically absorbed. The threat of absorption is always present:

The self is not being pegged in advance as a subject over against objects, but as involved essentially in a body which is pre-reflectively and non-thematically involved with others and in other things. [. . .] Because the body is ubiquitously but peripherally *along with* everything else in the field of experienced objects, it can be absorbed experientially in these objects. [. . .] The absorption of the experiencing body in the experienced object can proceed to the point where the *along-with* slips nonthematically into a magical or quasi-magical merging with the other, that being which officially (in Apollonian terms) one is not. The *along-with* slips into *being with* or *being in*.

(Wilshire 1982: 156–57)

The feeling of losing oneself into another, in love or in tenderness, or even to lose oneself in things, as when listening to music, gazing at a landscape or observing a natural phenomenon, is something that we have all experienced. This happens because both differentiation/separation and mimetic involvement with the other are a unique dynamic process in the development of the individual, comparable to the systole/diastole cycle of blood circulation. I become myself by differentiating myself from others, from a basic condition of mimetic absorption. The first differentiation is of course from the mother through a progressive and painful separation, which influences one's way of being in the world. John Bowlby (1988) has shown how many knots are tied on the attachment/separation/loss axis, making life unbearable for a lot of people. Bowlby considers the attachment to the mother from an ethological point of view, trying to go beyond the idea that dependency on the mother for nourishment is fundamental to the attachment process. He takes into consideration Konrad Lorenz's observations on behaviour patterns of ducklings: 'they develop a strong bond towards a specific maternal figure without the intermediation of food, since these small birds are not fed by their parents, but nourish themselves on insects' (Bowlby 1988: 24). At this point ethology turns to the concept of 'instinct', which, as Gregory Bateson has shown, is an 'explanatory principle, explaining everything that is needed to be explained by it' (Bateson 1972: 75). To proceed from here becomes more delicate. Perhaps the instinct of the ducklings following their mother is the same as Gurdulù who dissolves in a raft of ducks. Gurdulù does not 'believe he is a duck', but 'he believes to be the ducks.' His 'being the ducks' is pure presence, 'pre-reflexive and nonthematic', to use the words of Wilshire once again, therefore a basic part of his own being in the world.

At the other end of the spectrum we have the knight Agilulfo who creates his identity through a sequence of rigid separations. Agilulfo has a name and a story, and possesses a coat of shining armour that makes him identifiable by friends and enemies, but he doesn't have a body, and therefore doesn't exist. Not having a body makes him impermeable to mimetic absorptions, saving him from possible related emotional troubles, but at the same time it prevents him from growing: the dimension of becoming is blocked.

To conclude, being oneself is based in the end on being a body, and as such being subject to a dynamic flow between the conditions of being mimetically involved with others and being free from such conditions.

Possession and absence

At times the object takes the upper hand and submerges the subject – what Wilshire calls *mimetic engulfment* – blocking the dynamic possibility that is the only guarantee of a balanced relationship with the world. When Norman Bates commits his crimes in *Psycho*, Hitchcock's masterpiece of symbolic/visionary cinema, he is mimetically submerged by the figure of his dead mother. But Norman does much more. He takes on his mother's whole identity, wearing her clothes and her hair. It is the inverse process of losing oneself in the other in love, in aesthetical rapture and in transcendence. In that case, one's absorption in the other is a transport toward the other, a temporary but absolutely meaningful liberation from one's boundaries, or at least from boundaries self-attributed to oneself as a separate entity.

In love, this transport is toward the other as another person, therefore necessarily as a physical body. Accordingly, the mimetic absorption is mutual: 'You will be a single flesh.' In aesthetical rapture and in transcendence, it is toward the immaterial world where people for millennia had believed that spirits dwell. The central theme of all the mystical doctrines is the fusion of the individual with an absolute and total spiritual reality, whose meaning cannot be grasped within the limited categories available to our reason.

In a case such as Norman's, on the contrary, it is the other that takes over the individual, forcefully entering his body and taking abode. The mimetic absorption becomes an invasion, which forces the individual's boundaries, and cancels all the attributions of the self (purposes, feelings and projects).

Plato called 'divine folly' the state of possession by a divinity. Of the various forms of divine folly listed by Plato, through which 'the greatest goods are bestowed', the purifying folly has particular relevance to our discussion:

Sometimes, following evil and huge sufferings, effects of ancient resentments of the gods, this folly was generated in some of the people; once the future was foretold, it suggested to the appropriate authorities the way to avert other calamities, and they resorted to prayers and religious ceremonies. Once a way out from the evil of the moment was found for the one who was divinely mad and possessed, it also made those taking part in the purification and initiation rites immune in the present as well as in the future.

(Plato, *Phaedrus*: 244)

The purifying folly, called by Umberto Galimberti (1984) 'initiatic possession', is traditionally associated with the name of Dionysus. The origins of this mythological figure are complex and mysterious. They precede Hellenic civilization and vanish in the mists of time. The god of vegetation and fertility, of the phallus and of wine, of death and of rebirth, the stranger god, who came from somewhere else, has been compared to the Indian divinity Shiva, who plays the role of the destroyer, along with Brahma the creator and Vishnu the preserver.

Dionysus is particularly dear to the theatre: Greek tragedy evolved from ceremonies honouring this god. The name τραγωδία itself is derived from τράγος, the goat, symbolic of Dionysus, which was sacrificed in ceremonies dedicated to him. His is the first theatrical role endowed with an individual character. In the beginning only the choir or two dialoguing choirs existed. It is recounted that the legendary Thespis brought into the tragedy an actor who responded to the two choirs. Υποκριτής, a term subsequently used to designate any actor, means *the one who answers*. This actor played the role of Dionysus.

Another symbol for this god besides the goat and the phallus is the mask, and it is almost certain that theatrical masks originate from the Dionysian masks used in rites. But the mask of the god can also stand alone, without a body sustaining it: it was adored by the devoted who danced around a tree or pole where it was hung. 'The mask made the actor seem doubled in a strange way to the spectators: he was extraordinarily near and far at the same time' (Kerényi 1976).

For these very reasons the mask founds the theatre. Unlike what happens in rites, in which wearing a mask implies divine possession and consequently the annulment of the individual in a process of mimetic engulfment, the theatrical mask, the Persona, allows the regulation of mimetic involvement, in that it includes the concept of absence. The mask of Dionysus in the temple of Ikarion was a sign of the god's presence during his year of exile (within a two-year cycle; see Kerényi 1976).

At this point, person and mask, the two terms of the opening reflection, can be reconnected. I can be a person since as a physical body I am mimetically involved with others, but I can adjust this involvement by measuring the absence, as well as the presence, of the Other in me. I am perceived and recognized by others as a physical person, endowed with my own individuality and identity.

The theme of representation becomes central to our discussion at this point, which we will examine in the next section in terms of Jung's concept of Persona.

SOCIAL REPRESENTATIONS

> There are a great many men, but many more faces, because every man has quite a lot of them. There are people who wear a face for years, and it is natural that they wear it out; it becomes dirty, it thins out at the folds, it loses its shape as a travel-worn glove. They are simple, thrifty people; they don't change their face, they don't even clean it. 'It is still good,' they say, and who can convince them of the contrary? Of course, one might ask what they do with the others, since they have a whole stock of them. They put them aside. Their children will wear them. But it also happens that their dogs go out with those faces. Why not? A face is a face. Other people change their faces with exceptional rapidity, one after the other, and they wear them out. They think they have enough to last forever, but realize when they aren't even forty that they've got to the last one.
>
> (Rainer Maria Rilke, *The Notebooks of Malte Laurids Brigge*)

Consciousness and 'I'

In the previous section we focused on the body-self as the centre of the person, which develops its identity through the articulation of its mimetic involvements with the world, mirroring in the others' eyes. We have momentarily set aside the problem of the 'I', also because of a vague uneasiness linked to the consequences of the trend of thought, begun with Descartes, that sees in consciousness and in self-awareness the fundamental quality that confirms our existence. This paradigm has played an important role in the birth and development of modern thought. If the *I think* establishes the existence of the thinking human being, it follows that the mind is able to know itself and the world. An element of control and dominion is thus implicit: if I know the world I possess it, and I can mould it to meet my needs. The rational and conscious self becomes the absolute protagonist of the world stage, shadows dissolve and humanity proceeds toward its 'magnificent and progressive fates'. History has shown how this has been a great illusion. Never has humanity shown its dark side in such an arrogant and destructive way as in the present age of rapid scientific and technological advancement. The fact is that, in keeping with Freud's brilliant insight (already prophesied by the Romantics), even if we admit that the 'I' is *something*, it is not the master of its own house. According to Freud, the Ego ('I') is an essentially delicate element of the psychic apparatus, crushed as it is between the Es and the Super-Ego. All we do, say, and think, everything that determines who we are, is influenced, beyond our conscious will, by factors coming from territories extraneous to the 'I', whether they be the unknown seas of the Es or the pliers and shears of the Super-Ego.

Jung comes to an even more radical solution: for him the 'I' is:

> a complex of representations that for me is the centre of the field of my consciousness, and that seems to me to possess a high degree of continuity and identity with itself. Therefore I also speak of a complex of the 'I'. The complex of the 'I' is both a content and a condition of the consciousness, since a psychic element for me is conscious if referred to the complex of the 'I'. Nevertheless, since the 'I' is only the centre of the field of my consciousness, it is not identical to the totality of my psyche, but it is only a complex among so many complexes.
>
> (Jung 1921: 468)

This synthetic definition introduces two interesting areas of discussion that are well worth exploring. The first one pertains to the concept of representation. Jung uses this term in an extensive sense; in other words, he doesn't use it only in the sense intended by Saint Thomas of Aquino, for whom 'to represent something means to contain the simile of the thing' (*De Veritate*). For Jung, the problem of the object of representation is secondary. It can be an external object, therefore potentially knowable at a conscious level, but also an object of the inner reality, of the soul (*die Seele*, a term that Jung preferred to the more neutral and technical Psyche). In this case, the object is elusive and indefinable, and it can only be partially grasped by the consciousness, and consequently thematized. Representation can therefore be seen as an image, referring to something knowable, and as a symbol, referring to something not entirely knowable.

The consciousness, therefore, is not the protagonist, but a mere cipher in the immense theatre of the soul, crowded with images and symbols.

Indeed, images and symbols are somehow the substance of it. This oceanic theatre is defined by Jung as the *Selbst* (Self). In the *Selbst* Jung recognizes the basis of the life of the individual and of humanity, which ventures out into the domain of the sacred and the transcendent. The *Selbst* is in fact both individual and collective, as every individual soul participates in a heritage of images that belongs to the whole human kind, and that is expressed, at the highest levels, in poetic and spiritual terms. This concept of the *Selbst* brings us to the main idea of what Aldous Huxley has called, following Leibniz, the 'Philosophia Perennis', defining it as:

> A metaphysics that recognizes a divine Reality consubstantial to the world of things, of living creatures and of minds; a psychology that discovers in the soul something similar to divine Reality or even identical to it; an ethics that identifies man's final purpose as the knowledge of the immanent and transcendent Foundation of everything that exists.
>
> (Huxley 1945: 11)

In Jung's conception, aggregated nuclei emerge inside this undifferentiated ocean of images: floating islands such as the 'I' which is governed by the consciousness but actually is only partially conscious. The 'I' is 'the centre of the field of one's consciousness', and in this sense, although scaled down, the authority of the Cartesian *I Think* is recovered. However, the concept of the evidence of the 'I' as self-recognition of the individual is not specific to Western thought, but has an universal dimension. As the Upanishads say:

> In the beginning the universe was only the Atman (*the soul*) in the form of Puruša (*cosmic man*). Looking around him, he saw nothing but himself. The first thing he said was 'I am this!', and in this way the word 'I' was created. For this reason even today when someone is questioned the first thing he says is 'I am', then his name.
>
> (Brhadaranyaka Upanishad *IV*)

In the Indian myth, a chain of differentiations springs from the act of pronouncing the word 'I', which leads to the creation of the world and of humanity. But the identity of the universal soul with the individual soul remains; in fact the latter, after careful examination, reveals itself to be little more than an illusion. What is more, in turning to our second topic of discussion, in the sentence quoted from Jung an inkling of illusion is somehow present, if the election of the 'I' as 'centre of the field of consciousness' depends on the fact that 'it seems to possess a high degree of continuity and identity with itself'. This makes us think back to what was said in the first section about the need to construct the 'I' in the developmental process of differentiation, attributing to it a sense of continuity and identity, in the sense of Story and Name, and, accordingly, establishing some boundaries in the network of mimetic involvements in which our body-self is absorbed from birth, if not even before. The Italian psychologist Felice Perussia writes:

> It's a fact that the individual (every one of us, generally) tends to conceive the 'I' as a stable and durable substance. The choice to perceive it as constant is however mainly a postulate, allowing people to imagine the existence of an 'I', rather than the consequence of a proved continuity and stability of the same 'I' (as of the other). The person is not conceived as stable on the basis of a factual demonstration, because he mostly pays attention to the facts that show his own (and other people's) stability.
>
> (Perussia 2000: 141)

Even in its almost deceptive quality, the 'I' is necessary, for if its borders give way it can be catastrophic for the individual's very survival. For Jung this process has a name: possession. Unconscious psychic elements take the upper hand on the conscious self, and they force it to perform actions against its will. Jung calls these elements Archetypes, underlining their *numinous* nature, a term coined by the historian of religions Rudolf Otto to describe the ambivalent experience of the sacred *Mysterium Tremendum*; an experience that arouses veneration and fear. This term was explained by Jung as 'an essence or dynamic energy not originating from some arbitrary action of the will. On the contrary, this energy seizes and dominates the individual, who is always the victim of it rather than the creator' (Jung 1938–40: 17). Perhaps an extraordinarily ancient figure peeps out from behind the mother of Norman Bates, present in the most frightening fairytales and in the worst nightmares, as well as in myths: that of the Murderous Mother.

Person and self-identity

For Jung, however, there is another form of possession that doesn't cross the borders of insanity but blocks the process leading to the full development of human potentialities, which he calls the process of individuation:

Possession can be formulated as an identity of the personality of the 'I' with a variety of representations. A frequent case is the identity with the *Persona*, intended as a means of adaptation or a way of comparing oneself to the world. Almost every profession has one characteristic *Persona*. It is easy to observe these things today, given that people from the public sphere appear so often in newspapers. Society induces people to behave in a certain way, and those who have a professional role are forced to conform to these expectations. The only risk is to become identical to one's *Persona*: the teacher to his manual and the tenor to his voice. In this way the damage is done.

(Jung 1950: 120)

What is therefore his true character, his true personality? [. . .] In my opinion, the answer to this question is that such a person doesn't have a true character; that is, he is not *individual*, but *collective*, in harmony with the circumstances and general expectations. If he were individual he would always have the same character, despite differences in attitude. He would not be identical to the attitude assumed from time to time, nor would he be able to – or want to – prevent his individuality from expressing itself in any sort of situation. *In fact, a person is individual like all other human beings, but unconsciously so.* Through his complete identification with the attitude of the moment he deceives at least others, often even himself, as to his true character. He puts on a mask, aware that it corresponds on the one hand to his intentions, on the other to the demands and the opinions of his environment: at times the former prevails, at other times the latter. This mask, this attitude assumed ad hoc, I have called the *Persona*, from the name of the mask that the ancient actors wore.

(Jung 1921: 417)

The Persona is therefore also a 'complex of representations', that is, a group of images linked by a strong affective drive, which is a means of adapting to the world. In a certain sense it serves as an interface between the 'I' and the world. As the Jungian analyst Paolo Francesco Pieri writes: 'the *Persona* has the characteristic of something "already given" from the child's earliest experiences in the family (as the established place of roles), since its making can be attributed to the child's encounter with his father (emblematic of his relationships with others and with the world outside of the family)' (Pieri 1998: 538). In this association with the fatherly symbol, the Persona assumes a normative aspect besides that of necessity. If the father is the symbolic mediator of the relationship between the child and his social groups, it follows that the formation of the Persona, stretching out in the direction of the world of others (of the social world), is closely linked to what we could define as the interweaving of the mimetic identifications related to the fatherly area.

Unlike traditional societies, where roles, status and social hierarchies are rigidly fixed and unchangeable in time (as the caste system in traditional India), in our modern society a series of dynamic factors, connected with mobility, education, complexity of the job system, technological development and democratic political structures, allow a greater potential flexibility. Theoretically, it would be possible for every citizen to choose his own job and his proper place in the social context. Nevertheless, a lot of professions are handed down from father to child. We are not referring only to those professions involving a transmission of knowledge (such as the artisan, for instance, or the cook); rarely a parent who is a physician or a lawyer introduces his own child to medicine or to law. Instead, he would direct him to the right path, and perhaps even welcome him later to his own office to work at first as an employee, then as an associate, and finally, upon his own retirement, as the principal. In these cases, the family tradition imposes a persistence of the Persona that passes from one generation to the next, exactly like the descendants of kings. The regal figure exists apart from the particular individual who embodies it, and every sovereign is bound, from birth, to conform to systems of behaviour that regulate the appearances and the manifestations of it in a total and absolute way. When this Persona collapses, there is no other choice for the person than to keep playing his part (to keep his mask), even in front of the guillotine, or to shatter into pieces, cancelling himself, as is the case with the Last Emperor of China, masterfully narrated in Bernardo Bertolucci's film.

But, returning to the physicians and lawyers (and also the notaries, politicians, executives and actors), it is curious to notice that the transmission occurs from father to son or at times from father to daughter – almost never from mother to daughter. I could speculate that in the symbolic universe in which we are immersed the maternal galaxy leads to the internal world, to the dream and the rêverie, while the paternal one embraces the external world, the things and issues between people. But this doesn't mean that the Persona is a masculine prerogative: if its structure is made by the encounter with the father, its form depends on the encounter with the others. For teenagers (male or female), it can be necessary to assume an opposite Persona to the one already given by the family tradition, for the purpose of underlining their separation and escaping from a mimetic engulfment that threatens the formation of what is perceived as their own identity (the power to say 'I', as the cosmic man of the Upanishads).

According to Erik H. Erikson (1968), adolescents are facing a crisis in which old values and new chances are conflicting. They search for new identifications with peers or with leading figures outside the family, in an incessant effort to 'define, redefine and over-define' themselves and others in constant comparisons. In a striking apologue, the American cartoonist Jules Feiffer (1968) shows us a young fellow in perfect high school clothes (tennis shoes, jacket, and a book under his arm) saying:

> Since the time I was a child I didn't want to be me. I wanted to be Billie Widdledon. And Billie Widdledon didn't even like me. I walked like him. I talked like him. And I enrolled in the same high school as he did. It was then that Billie Widdledon changed. He started to hang around with Herby Vandeman. He walked like Herby Vandeman. He talked like Herby Vandeman. I began to get confused. I tried walking and talking like Billie Widdledon who walked and talked like Herby Vandeman. And I realized that Herby Vandeman walked and talked like Joe Haverin and Joe Haverin walked and talked like Corky Sabinson. So I had to walk and to talk like Billie Widdledon's imitation of Herby Vandeman imitating Joe Haverin who was trying to walk and talk like Corky Sabinson. And who do you think Corky Sabinson was imitating? Among everyone he chose that idiot Kenny Wellington. That idiot who walks and talks like me.
>
> (Feiffer 1968)

This little sketch describes a chain of mimetic identifications that goes in a vicious circle. The laborious search for identity turns into a game of masks. On the other hand Jung himself warns us:

> Conscious personality is a more or less arbitrary segment of the collective psyche. It consists of a sum of psychic facts felt as personal. The personal attribute expresses the exclusive affiliation to a determined person. A consciousness that is *only* personal affirms with a certain anxiety its right of ownership and of priority to its own contents, and it tries to make a complete entity of it. But the contents that are not framed in this entity are neglected and forgotten or removed and disowned. This is also a kind of self-education, but too arbitrary and too violent. It requires the sacrifice of too many universally human things for an ideal image to which we would like

to conform. [. . .] I have called *Persona* this segment often drawn with so much effort from the collective psyche. [. . .]

Only because the *Persona* is a more or less accidental or arbitrary segment of the collective psyche can we fall into the trap of considering it, even *in toto*, as something individual; but, as the name itself implies, it is only a mask of the collective psyche, a mask that simulates individuality, that makes others believe that whoever puts it on is individual, while it is only a part played in the theatre in which the collective psyche speaks.

(Jung 1928: 154–5)

To recapitulate, the conscious 'I' attributes a continuity to its own physical body that defines it as an individual, and manifests itself through masks suited for different contexts. The Persona is a complex structure of mimetic images that people build as a membrane between themselves and the external world, with protective and adaptive functions. The material of which this structure is made cannot be defined as individual, as it is formed with the expectations, rules, traditions, images, behaviour systems and values that belong to the collective sphere. The protective function of the Persona has a double quality: on the one hand it allows us not to be excluded from the groups with which we interact, as our performances are approved and shared by others. On the other hand, it allows the self to maintain control over a universe of relationships that threatens to mimetically submerge us. Without the Persona, the self would be naked and without skin, prey to the storms of the external world. But if the self gets lost in the Persona, and bases his own identity on it, he loses the possibility of becoming a true individual, sacrificing 'too many universally human things'.

Social masks

The reflections on this concept of the Persona as social mask bring us back to the questions outlined at the beginning of the first section, and lead us to a point of view that, from sociologist Erving Goffman's challenging ideas, has not only influenced much scientific thought on social life, but also common thought: that of the society as theatre. Shakespeare had already introduced this theme with the famous lines of Jacques in *As You Like It*: 'All the world's a stage, and all the men and women merely players. They have their exits and their entrances, and one man in his time plays many parts' (II, vii).

Goffman analyses social interactions in terms of a central idea: that the presentation of self which all of us perform in front of others has some rules that can be described as dramatic. These rules are particularly visible in more organized social contexts, as in public ritualistic events. In events such as marriages and funerals, it is necessary to conform to stylized behaviours dictated by the traditions of the group in which the event happens. Unconventional behaviours, such as laughing at a funeral or getting drunk at a wedding, are also somehow included in a possible script. The same thing happens in institutional contexts or in work groups. But Goffman's study goes further. The fact is that it is not possible to ignore others: the freedom to express ourselves cannot be total. According to Goffman, when an individual appears before others, his actions influence the definition that is assigned to the situation:

> At times the individual acts in an entirely calculated way, expressing himself only in such a way as to give the kind of impression that has the probability of soliciting the particular reaction that he is interested in getting from others. On other occasions he acts by calculation, even though he is only relatively aware of it, and at times he intentionally and consciously expresses himself in a determined way above all because the tradition of his group or social status demands it, in order not to get a particular reaction (aside from a vague acceptance or approval). Finally, at times the implicit traditions of the individual's role help him to give a very precise impression, even though he is not trying, consciously or unconsciously, to create such impressions.
>
> (Goffman 1959: 16)

Even though he states the possibility that theatrical strategies of action, which are aimed at creating an appearance that can be acknowledged by others and can influence the general perception of the context, are only partially deliberate and conscious, Goffman focuses his analysis on those situations in which the presentation of self is deliberately aimed at personal advantage:

> A presentation can be defined as the whole activity developed by a participant in a determined occasion and directed somehow to influence any of the participants.
>
> (Goffman 1959: 26)

I wonder if it is enough to include a shade of deliberateness in the concept of representation in order that the sense of deception and fraud is insinuated. For a long time the acting profession has been looked upon with suspicion. In the Middle Ages the idea of deception in drama was linked to the Great Deceiver, and actors were buried in desecrated ground. Perhaps we find it difficult to accept that someone is paid to do what we all do every day out of necessity – play a part.

Goffman examines in detail the strategies that people set in motion to present themselves in social interactions, and continues using the theatrical metaphor to list the tools of these performances: the *setting* (that is, the theatrical scenery), the personal *façade* (referring to external aspects, such as costumes and make-up, and to the types of behaviours – the acting style), and the *routines* (the scripts to be respected). The staging is often sustained by a group of people that Goffman calls the *équipe*, defining it as 'a group of individuals who must collaborate to maintain a certain definition of the situation' (in theatre this is the company of actors).

Such a line of thought can easily be debased in a tendency to conform to the 'correct way to act', the possibility of being successful in life. 'How to make friends and influence people' was the advertising slogan (and perhaps also the title) of countless booklets that showed people the road to happiness and success (mocked by Bob Dylan in his Tombstone Blues: 'a fantastic/collection of stamps/to win friends and influence his uncle'). Today, important political parties expect their key members to undergo training on image management.

In fact, the situation is far more complex. Of course, we often use conscious strategies to construct appearance with the intention to produce a desired effect on others. But the mimetic interweaving through which the Persona is formed is to a large extent unconscious, and can also lead us in the opposite direction. However, Goffman reminds us that it is not always easy to prepare a suitable presentation, and mentions various forms of 'loss of control' on stage by the actor:

> Indeed, an actor can incidentally communicate incapability, incorrectness, or insolence, momentarily losing control of his own muscles. He can stumble, tumble, fall, yawn, make a blunder, scratch himself or pass wind; he can also accidentally bump into another actor. Secondly, an actor can give the impression that he is either too interested or not interested enough in the interaction by stammering, forgetting his lines, appearing nervous, guilty or embarrassed, breaking into inappropriate laughter, or expressing anger or other emotions that momentarily hinder the interaction. Finally, an actor's performance can reveal the effects of inadequate stage directions. The staging can be messy, it can have been arranged for a different

presentation, or it can change during the action; unexpected factors can result in miscalculating the timing of an actor's entrances or exits, or can cause embarrassing pauses during the performance.

(Goffman 1959: 64–65)

It seems that in order to survive in a basically hostile world, it is necessary to build a strong Persona (or more than one), removing, in a way that Jung defines as arbitrary and violent, the intimate, universally human qualities of the individual, connected to sensibility, feelings and emotions. These qualities exist in the soul (in the psyche) of everyone as mimetic potentiality, and can be strengthened or inhibited according to individual experience. In some subcultures based on particularly rigid Personae, the expression of feelings is strictly forbidden. The late Giovanni Falcone,[2] recognized as one of the most acute observers of the Mafia phenomenon besides his fame as a great man of law, observes:

A *Mafioso* who shows signs of psychological uneasiness and therefore insecurity, risks being definitively silenced. [. . .] This helps us to understand why the *Mafioso* doesn't speak, why he never allows emotions or feelings to slip out.

(Falcone 1991: 52)

A person who expresses emotions and feelings outside of specific circumstances in which this is tolerated shows weakness and vulnerability, and he can turn out to be a risk for an organization founded on cast-iron rules of dominance and submission and on the code of silence. On the other hand, Falcone underlines how it is often the breaking in – sometimes unexpectedly – of the affective and emotional world that triggers processes of transformation inducing many so-called men of honour to turn their backs on the organization and the rigid culture that sustains it.

Of course, this is an extreme example. It is true, however, that it is easy for all of us to perceive the signals coming from those around us as a sum of demands, pressures, obligations and prayers that influence our behaviour in conformity with the rules. These rules are not always entirely known and understood, but we must adjust to them in order to construct a mimetic Persona that reflects the codes and values (implicit or explicit) of a community that grants us the authorization to exist.

If this is a challenge of survival, not everyone is able to face it. At times I perceive a correspondence between my Persona, modelled by and adapted to the others' vision of me, and my identity defined by the history of my body-self (what Paul Schilder 1935 calls my body-image). In this case my conscious 'I' feels separate, exiled from what the others perceive and accept as myself, an identity that seems false to me. This is what R. D. Laing (1959) calls 'the false Ego system', in which people 'perceive their self, whether it be called internal, true or real, as separate from all of their observable activity'. The feeling is therefore that one just acts, not being really present in the world. Laing defines this situation as *schizoid condition*, and considers it a possible herald of insanity.

Traps of identity

We have mentioned two extreme conditions in which identity becomes a trap wherein our potential for developing and accomplishing ourselves as individuals is caught. The first one is the possession by the Persona: in it the 'I' identifies with the Persona to the extent that it transfers all of the characteristic attributions of its identity into it. This transfer also takes place in the second condition, the *false Ego system*. In this case, however, the 'I' separates from the Persona, and 'assuming the "I" to be unrelated to it, it removes itself from the real world and it faces exclusively abstract and therefore inactive or ineffective possibilities' (Pieri 1998: 52).

But there is another condition in this threefold game: when consciousness and body-self are fused to the point that they create an implosive form of identity, closed in on itself. The Persona is out of the person's reach. Access to the world is denied because it can only be granted in the presence of what could be defined as a protective mediation, hiding and revealing at the same time. Considered as a feature of social relationships, the Persona composes and reassembles the mimetic expectations that connect one person to another; in this sense it maintains distance while at the same time allowing communication and contact to take place. Without this interface with the world, the individual cannot control the emotional–mimetic exchanges between himself and others, and cannot bear relationships, except mimetically saturated ones, such as dependency relationships (or, in its more extreme form, relationships in which love and hate are mingled).

We can try to summarize what has been said in the last few pages with a diagram. In Figure 1.1, identity is represented as the place where 'I', body-self and Persona (considered also as multiple Personae) overlap. Each of these elements has an edge that both separates it from and connects it with the outside (the others – the world). Imbalanced conditions are represented by the intersections of any two elements, excluding the third one.

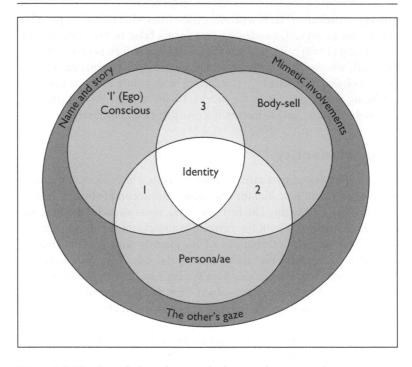

Figure 1.1 Identity as balance between body, consciousness and appearance

Segment 1 represents *Possession*. The 'I' identifies completely with the Persona or with the Personae that one acts on the stage of life. I would like once again to quote Shakespeare's Jacques, with his metaphor of the world as a stage, where 'one man in his time plays many parts':

> His acts being seven ages. At first the infant,
> mewling and puking in the nurse's arms.
> Then the whining schoolboy with his satchel
> And shining morning face, creeping like snail
> Unwillingly to school. And then the lover,
> Sighing like furnace, with a woeful ballad
> Made to his mistress' eyebrow. Then, a soldier,
> Full of strange oaths, and bearded like the pard,
> Jealous in honour, sudden, and quick in quarrel,
> Seeking the bubble reputation
> Even in the cannon's mouth. And then the justice,
> In fair round belly with good capon lined,

With eyes severe and beard of formal cut,
Full of wise saws and modern instances;
And so he plays his part. The sixth age shifts
Into the lean and slippered pantaloon,
With spectacles on nose and pouch on side,
His youthful hose, well saved, a world too wide
For his shrunk shank, and his big, manly voice,
Turning again towards childish treble, pipes
And whistles in his sound. Last scene of all,
That ends this strange, eventful history,
In second childishness and mere oblivion,
Sans teeth, sans eyes, sans taste, sans everything.

(As You Like It, II; vii)

In this vision (which actually the same comedy denies, as well as the whole of Shakespeare's works), it is impossible to rebel against the mask. The dimension of freedom is totally denied (which is the equivalent in relational terms of what is represented by creativity at an intra-personal level).

Segment 2 represents *Exile* (of the 'I'). Even here the Persona has taken the upper hand, incorporating the whole mimetic–emotional side of the personal history, to the detriment of the 'I', that feels distant from the mask that he wears on the stage of life, as well as from their own emotions: the 'I' watches itself living:

Things happen to the other, to Borges. I walk around Buenos Aires and stop, perhaps by now mechanically, to look at the arch of an entrance-way and at a door that opens onto a courtyard; I have news of Borges through the mail and I see his name in a list of teachers and in a biographical dictionary. I like hourglasses, maps, XVIII century prints, coffee and Stevenson's prose; the other shares these preferences, but in a vain way that changes them into the attributes of an actor. It would be exaggerated to say that our relationship is hostile: I live, I let myself live, so that Borges can conjure his literature, and this justifies me.

(Borges 1960)

Segment 3 represents *Absence*. This is the opposite of the other two: while in possession and exile the remarkable aspect is the predominance of the Persona, albeit with different features, in absence it is the lack of this precious (if used well) diaphragm that makes the individual incapable of having interpersonal relationships, and incapable of filtering messages (including emotional ones) from others. This results in the painful feeling of being 'skinless', flung onto the stage of life without a role or a script to act.

To remain within the dramatic metaphor, we could say that the first condition is equivalent to the actor's total identification with the character. Of course, this results in successful performances but tends to limit the expressive possibilities of the actor, who keeps playing the same sort of role, and ends up bringing the role with him offstage, even into his private life. This actor will find it difficult to change roles and dramatic genre, and in the end he will find himself confined to an identity that is not his own. Another condition is that of total separation. The actor plays his role in a technically precise way, using gestures and tones of voice which meet the public's expectations perfectly, but he 'lacks soul'; he doesn't live in the character and he doesn't bring the character to life. His fate is that of coldness and mediocrity, until a crisis arrives unexpectedly, confusing his sense of identity. The third condition is the impossibility to go on stage. This actor is condemned to remain in the wings forever, or, if he is pushed on stage, he will probably suffer an attack of what is called stage fright in theatre, and will not be able to act at all. (People would say, 'He can't play', where 'to play' can mean both children's play and theatre acting; that is why Brook, in his reflections on the nature of theatre, says 'A play is play').

Perhaps identity exists and lives the life of humans with the aim of its complete realization only in virtue of a fragile balance, in continuous transformation, among body, consciousness and appearance. This issue is particularly remarkable if we look at it within the frame of the historic social sea-changes in which we are involved. In traditional societies, personal identity is something which is assigned to people from their birth, but in our time, defined by Giddens (1991), we are merged with an increasingly complex web of levels of experience and relationships, involving opportunities and risks. The old patterns of identity are broken and a new concept is required, seeing identity as a never-ending project of search. Giddens's viewpoint still considers the existence of a core self, able to be the author of the project, by generating a continuous self-reflexive process. Other scholars, like Kenneth Gergen (1991), believe that the loss of this point of reference is an unavoidable step in the shifting between modern age and postmodern, toward which we run at astonishing speed:

If it is not individual 'I' who create relationships, but relationships that create the sense of 'I', then 'I' cease to be the center of success or failure, the one who is evaluated well or poorly.

(Gergen 1991: 157)

Gergen makes an attempt to create a new vocabulary for this condition; he speaks of *multiphrenia, pastiche personality* and *ersatz being*. Is it the ultimate loss of a would-be ethos of the human being? Gergen stresses the positive potentiality of this condition, as an 'invitation to Carnival', but there's still an emerging question: is there any difference between fully living it, investing in its intrinsic dimension of freedom, and a mere being subjected to it? And if so, which are the basic criteria to establish the difference? Ascribing meaning to experience is an accomplishment that needs a subject to be the agent of it; the idea of personal identity, though overwhelmed by a fundamental relativism involving the notion of reality itself and therefore submitted to a radical metamorphosis, emerges as a necessity. Yet, it cannot be conceived but in the form of a quest. In the next chapters, we will try to explore drama as a place where this quest can have room, through languages, images and metaphors, and, above all, through an encounter of human beings.

But before discussing this matter further, let me play a variation on the theme of the mask, which is the subject of the next section.

BEYOND THE MASK

> Maya, Maya,
> All the world is but a play:
> Be thou the joyful player.
> (Robin Williamson, *Maya*)

Persona's collapse

In Marcel Schwob's novel *The King with the Golden Mask* (1892), a situation is portrayed in which the mask is mandatory: 'Once the city was governed by princes who did not cover their faces; but since then a long succession of masked kings had come to the throne. No one had ever seen their face, and even the priests didn't know why.'

All the people living at court or nearby are compelled to wear masks consistent with their role: jesters, priests, soldiers and concubines. All of them take part in a performance focused on the protagonist, following the rules of public presentations in detail, as described by Goffman: the *staging* (the scene of the court); the personal *façade* (the mask, of course, but also attitudes and rules of behaviour); the *routines* (the rhythms of court life). Everyone cooperates to maintain the definition of the situation: they act as an *équipe*. The whole thing is balanced and perfect: the action revolves around the king, marked by his gold mask. Nevertheless, at some point a new element is introduced, setting the story in motion. A blind beggar comes to the king's court, without a mask, and tells the king about his perceptions:

> 'Listen: you are the king, but you don't know your subjects. These on my left are the jesters – I hear them laughing; these on my right are the priests – I hear them crying; and I can tell that the faces of these women are drawn in a grimace.'
>
> So the king turned toward those the beggar called jesters, and he found the caring black masks of the priests; he turned toward those the beggar called priests, and found the smiling masks of the jesters; he lowered his eyes toward his women, seated in a semicircle, and their faces looked beautiful to him.

The king therefore sends the beggar away, accusing him of lying. But a doubt has started creeping into his mind: the doubt that things, and even his very identity, are different from what the eyes see. One night he secretly leaves the palace for the outside world, searching for a denial or a confirmation to his presentiments. The figure of the king running away from court life enclosed within the palace walls to see the world, and to begin a quest for knowledge that will provoke profound changes in him, is a recurring theme in stories that narrate the hero's journey – a journey of transformation and renewal (see Campbell 1949). Among these is the legend of Buddha. As it is recounted, an oracle announces to king Suddhodana that an extraordinary future awaits his child, prince Siddhartha. If he succeeded to the throne, he would become the greatest king in history, but if he chose the path of asceticism, he would become a great Master. He would discover the sufferings of the world and the way to put an end to them. Suddhodana, worried about losing his child and heir to the throne, orders that the palace be provided with all sorts of pleasure and amusements, and that any trace of pain and suffering, even the smallest wrinkle on the face of a woman, be eliminated. So the future Buddha spends his youth happily and innocently, unaware that illness, old age and death exist in the world. But one day, while walking in the city, something goes awry in the controlled performance, and the prince sees an old man, a sick man and a corpse. This experience changes the prince's life to the extent that one night, prey to an implacable restlessness, he leaves the palace and its pleasures to go and see the world.

The king of Schwob's novel returns instead to the palace, but only after having discovered that under his own golden mask hides a 'pale, swollen face, covered with scabs and filthy sores': his true face was that of a leper. This intolerable revelation completely upsets the king's life. The mask had covered a repugnant horror for all those years, but more dreadful than the illness itself is deception unveiled. If the Persona I have worn until the present covered a part of me that I didn't know and of which I am ashamed, then what sense can the world that I have known till now have, once I have discovered the secret? All the values, the feelings, the meanings of things and people must be redefined, but the struggle to redefine them is an uneven one, and I can easily succumb. The collapse of the Persona is, according to Jung, 'a leaning out over that psychic abyss in which manifold ambivalent images are given' (Pieri 1998: 541). The greatest dangers ensuing from this collapse are:

> the regressive reconstruction of the *Persona*, that is, the risk of an escapist attitude towards a wealth of different configurations, which involves the 'I' reassuming the *Persona* as a protective armour; the shattering of the psyche, that is, the risk of a shipwreck of the 'I' in the constitutive ambivalence of all the figurations of the collective unconscious; the inflation of the 'I', that is, the risk of a falsifying identity, by which the 'I' assumes the role of specific configurations of the collective unconscious in their most seductive but also childish aspects (the absolutely tragic figure of the prophet and that of the tragicomic fanatical disciple of a prophet).
>
> (ibid.)

The king doesn't take any of these possible paths. The shame and bitterness of his discovery are so great that he decides to dramatically unmask all the people responsible for the performance:

> So the king sat upon the black throne and declared: 'I have struck the gong to tell you something important. The beggar was telling the truth. All of you here have deceived me. Remove the masks from your faces.'
>
> You could hear arms, clothing, weapons shake with fear. Then, slowly, all the people gathered there took off their masks.

Then the king with the golden mask turned toward the priests and saw fifty laughing faces with little squinty eyes; and, turning toward the jesters, he saw fifty pale faces hollowed by sadness, with eyes reddened from insomnia; and lowering his eyes toward the semicircle of women, he sneered. . .because their faces were full of boredom and ugliness and painted with stupidity. [. . .]

And the king removed his gold mask. A cry went up from those who saw him, for the brazier's pink flame illuminated the pale scabby skin of a leper.

(ibid.)

At the climax of the tragic unveiling, in which the world shows its ominous side behind the mask, the king announces: 'I won't be deceived by the appearances of this world anymore, and I will direct my gaze toward dark things.' Saying this, he sticks the hooks of his own mask in his eyes, blinding himself, as Oedipus did (in Sophocles's *Oedipus Rex*) with the gold buckles taken from his mother/wife's dresses. Oedipus also receives from a blind clairvoyant the revelation that behind the visible world that he has built around himself is concealed another world, full of horror and dismay; that behind his mask of wise king of Thebes hides the ambiguous face of a parricide.

Mask and truth

Although unaware, Oedipus breaks a rule crucial for the survival of humanity itself: he has turned a metaphor into an act of reality. All of us may have had a moment of discouragement at some time in our lives when we have expressed the strong desire to die. But from expressing such a thought to the act of suicide itself there is a great distance. 'I feel like dying' or 'I could kill you' belong to the same metaphoric world of 'I am in heaven' or 'I am bursting with joy', in which the meaning of the words is not to be understood in the literal sense, but as a synthetic allusion to another deeper meaning. So 'to take one's father's place' might be a metaphor of the process of personal growth, with an extension that goes from 'taking over the family firm' (as the professionals already mentioned): to 'assuming an adult role of responsibility', to 'eliminating my father image' (setting oneself free from a mimetic engulfment by the fatherly image to create new role possibilities). Oedipus takes concrete action instead. He takes his father's place by killing him and then joining with his father's wife.

On the other hand, 'taking the father's place' is only a specific case of the more general one of mimetically construing ourselves in comparison with others, of our taking the other's place. This process occurs only within a network of authorizations. Only if I am authorized to grow by a *good enough mother* (see Winnicott) can I take my first steps toward separating from her to find new models of identification; in other words, to open new mimetic channels with the world. This involves, in turn, other forms of authorization, not only from figures of authority (above all the father), but also from peers (friends and companions), from institutions (school, church, and so on) and from other figures of attachment (the partner, the affective network). Only by constructing an identity that I consider suitable enough can I authorize myself to be the master of my own destiny; to use another dramatic metaphor, to be the author of the script that I act out every day.

This possibility is not given to Sophocles's Oedipus, as it is not given to the man/actor described seven centuries later by Epictetus (p. 11). His destiny is to wear the masks that he meets along his path, never knowing the truth until the tragic end in which all the masks collapse.

At this point the theme of truth hiding behind the mask comes forcefully into play. This is a particularly delicate theme, first of all because the concept of truth is a normative concept. We consider truth as equivalent to being. According to Aristotle: 'To deny what is and to affirm what is not, is falsehood; whether to affirm what is and to deny what is not, is the truth' (*Metaphysics*). In this case the problem lies in establishing the criteria of correspondence that can only be determined by an authority figure. In the modern world, this task is usually assigned to science, for which one of the principal criteria of truth is conformity to experience, in its rigid, structured and repeatable form of the experiment (though everyone knows how easy it is to falsify an experiment). In the case in question, the tautological aspect of the dichotomy of truth/falsehood is evident: truth is what it is behind the mask – whatever it may be. The mask is therefore a form of appearance that hides, conceals, and deceives. But this is perhaps a good thing, since what lurks behind appearance is always something horrible, which we could not bear to see.

This seems to be the case for the king of Schwob's novel, whose miserable fate is that of a vagabond, even though, as for Oedipus, his death is noble: 'He has taken off all the masks, of gold, of leprosy and of flesh.' Similarly, Oedipus 'disappeared in an almost celestial calm: a superhuman amazement' (Sophocles, *Oedipus at Colonus*).

The middle course

So it is for the young prince Siddhartha, who discovers how behind the masks of joy and pleasure hides the unavoidability of pain: aging, sickness, and death. Far from his father's palace, the future Buddha removes his regal clothing, cuts off his hair, sends away his horse and gets ready to follow the path of the spirit according to custom – a path of abstinence, fasting, and mortification of the flesh:

> At mealtime he ate only a single jujube fruit, a single sesame seed, a single grain of rice, since he wanted to reach the other shore of the cycle of rebirths, the one with endless bounds.
>
> (Asvaghosa, *The Deeds of the Buddha*, XII: 96)

But the mortification of the flesh does not produce the desired results:

> How can the restless one, exhausted from hunger, thirst and mortifications, whose mind can hardly function from fatigue, be able to reach the result that the mind has to reach?
>
> (ibid., XII: 103)

So Siddhartha, after six long years of self-denial and self-torture, decides to start eating again, and accepts a bowl of milk and rice from a young girl. At this moment, the process that will bring him to Enlightenment begins.

This episode helps us to understand why Buddhism has constantly defined itself 'The Middle Course'. Between the total surrender to the world of the senses and the negation of the body, Buddha chooses a reasonable intermediate position. In the same way, the world vision of Enlightenment takes us along a path that runs midway between reality and illusion. Life, as it is experienced by sentient beings, is made of pain and suffering, due to the basic ignorance of the fact that everything we perceive as existing is fundamentally an illusory appearance: a life of *conditioned co-production*, in which people and objects don't exist in and of themselves, but only as mutual relationships. We cling to these things for survival: emotional attachments, material objects, our physical body, even our identity, regardless of the fact that everything is non-permanent. Everything is destined to end and to be consumed, or to turn into something different. The theme of illusion (the world as a dream) was recurrent in Indian philosophy even before Buddha's time, and it was later included in the Vedanta doctrine that also influenced Schopenhauer. The wise man therefore distances himself from this game of masks (the mask of attachment that hides the mask of suffering, which is itself a pretence) to face the dimension of the Void (Sunyata).[3] But everyday reality is not abolished: Buddha, after having reached Enlightenment, doesn't choose the way of isolation and contemplation, but returns among the people to preach. The world of conditioned co-production is not pure illusion: we are part of it, with our body and our emotions. We know that it is just a matter of acting, but in the meanwhile we act. We laugh and we cry, but above all we practise being-with-others (the *mit-dasein* of the analytical-existential tradition; see Biswanger 1921–41), developing the most important virtue – Compassion (*Karuna*). Through *Karuna*, the wise person participates in the world, welcoming the joy and pain of others and contemplating into them the unique essence to which we all belong, that is a universal soul (the nature of Buddha in all sentient beings). In the words of a great Italian poetess:

> In the difficult commandment: Love others as you love yourself,
> The *as* should be read as *because*. BECAUSE
> The other – the others
> They are all Yourself.
>   (Elsa Morante, *The World Saved by Kids*, 1968)

In the meantime, wise people are aware that it is only a matter of a masquerade: they are able to be both involved and detached. In this sense they are like the actor who, although he/she knows that what is happening on stage is only a performance, cries real tears and laughs with true laughter. 'Attention!' sing the mynah birds in the woods of Pala island (in Aldous Huxley's novel *Island*), as a constant reminder that the world is an illusion, and attaching oneself to it is foolish and the cause of suffering. But immediately after they sing 'Karuna!'

Chapter 2

Threshold

THE RITE OF AUTHORIZATION

> 'What an excellent idea!' Said Wilhelm, 'In a society in which no one fakes, in which people follow only their own feeling, neither grace nor happiness can survive for a long time, but, on the other hand, in a society in which everybody pretends, they never show themselves. It is not bad therefore that we deliberately start with a pretence, to be then, under the mask, sincere as we want.'
>
> (Johann Wolfgang Goethe, *The Novitiate of Wilhelm Meister*)

The permission to exist

In our meanderings among the various masks, we have touched upon the Oedipus myth. The central part of this myth concerning the protagonist's personal destiny has become, thanks to Freud and psychoanalysis, one of the stories that has influenced modern thought to the greatest extent. The theme of *taking the father's place*, developed in the story of Oedipus through the transgression of some of the basic rules of society, has been used as a metaphor for understanding the bonds of children with their own parents, bonds that are ineluctable and potentially pathological, in a precarious equilibrium between desire and reality. On the other hand, Winnicott, speaking of the unconscious fantasies of adolescence, reminds us that 'if the child is to become an adult, then this transformation must take place over the dead body of an adult'.

In more general terms, we can place this theme in a wider framework concerning the relationship with an authority who can grant or deny the permission to exist. As mentioned in the previous chapters, in order to exist and to define ourselves as individuals, we need to be mirrored and defined by others. One of the most subtly penetrating myths of the Modern

Age comes to mind, that of Robinson Crusoe. Alone in a strange place, with no one to speak to but his own thoughts, Robinson reconstructs his identity as master of the island, by means of his civilizing virtues of *homo faber*. But even he, after a while, needs another person to confirm his own identity. It is of course the matter of an Other with neither name nor story – the savage, who can only reflect back our superiority. He is therefore necessary.

From the Other I receive the fundamental confirmation of my existence. Moreover, from the Other, in his particular configuration as Authority (from the Latin *auctoritas*, legitimacy, that has the same root as *auctor*, author, but also founder) I receive authorization to go along my way. 'The permission to exist,' writes Perussia, 'is the acceptance of spontaneity. It is the activation of the person in the sense of facilitating their natural disposition to be actor-author. It is developing, or rediscovering, the natural ability to accept or to refuse the proposals of the world' (2000: 275). Oedipus has not received this authorization. He is particularly gifted, which allows him to resolve enigmas (except his own), but he cannot choose. He carries out the deadly prophecy of the oracle – that the son shall kill his own father – but totally unaware. He runs away from Corinth to avoid submitting to the prophecy, but it is precisely this escape that allows the crime to occur and the fate to come true. He will take his father's place, becoming actually king of Thebes, but the substitution is illegitimate.

The permission to stand in

It is important for this discussion to underline the fact that the myth of Oedipus, with its themes of masks and unmasking, taking another's place and authority, was passed down to us not just through narrative but particularly through the theatre. Its themes deal specifically with human relationships, on which the theatre as an activity of the human community is founded. Writes Wilshire:

> Oedipus stands in illicitly for the authority. If to stand in for an authority licitly is to be authorized, to stand in illicitly must be condemned and defiled. In the theatre event the community stands in licitly for Oedipus' illicit standing in, and thereby transcends the defilement in the very act of participating in it vicariously. The community of individuals authorizes itself as a community and as individuals.
>
> (Wilshire 1982: 59)

To *stand in for* is, according to Wilshire, a basic feature of human relationships: the making of individual identity through a continuous oscillating movement between mimetic involvements and disengagement from them. The nature of the theatre is one of performance and of interpretation. The actor stands in for the character, and the character stands in for each member of the audience. But the actor is not entirely and permanently the character, as we are not Oedipus, even if we mimetically find parts of Oedipus inside of us. The actor performs the character, and in a peculiar way becomes him, but not totally. In the performance an approach to the character is implicit, which is mimetic recognition, but also interpretation. To interpret means to lead the other-from-myself to forms that are compatible with the codes and the constructs that regulate my interactions with the world, and are therefore communicable. Performance/ interpretation is presence/absence, possession and distance. The spectator, who enters into a mimetic relationship (of identification and separation) with the actor who performs/interprets the character, in turn sees himself in that performance/interpretation, thus giving it meaning. An analogous process happens in life. Continues Perussia:

> The game of actions and reactions is organized around a process of continuous definition of the events that can be ascribed to some individuals, both in terms of their (and our) actions and in terms of their (and our) reactions. Thus life, from birth to death, is a continuous performance in which everyone plays endless parts, eliciting endless feelings. Even here, it is a question of representation in both a transitive and an intransitive sense. Representations (as interpretations, in the individual) concern the way of living the actions and giving an internal resonance to them. Representations (as performances on the stage of the world) concern the way of dramatizing, or concretising, our own experiences in actions.
>
> (Perussia 2000: 151)

I construct myself as a person through the interplay of performance/ interpretation. Theatre provides an opportunity for this kind of play to be declared and openly enacted, through the sharing of some simple rules between actor and spectator. The first is the acceptance of the *as if* paradox that we can call, to use Coleridge's genial expression once again, 'the deliberate suspension of disbelief'. What happens on the stage is not real in the sense in which my dog, my table or my colleagues are real for me, but I can and I must act as if it were. This is true for both the actor, who mainly gives what Perussia calls an active performance, and for the spectator, who undergoes primarily mimetic identification. The 'as if' paradox is the door that allows us to cross the borders between the world and the 'world'. We will return later to the theme of 'as if' as a factor triggering the creative process. The main point here is to clarify the core of the matter: in the theatrical event the potentiality of standing in for (and accordingly of performance/interpretation) is collectively and legitimately authorized, in all possible directions:

> The shimmering fictional character is the locus through which the actor is given back to himself through the audience, and the members of the audience are given back to themselves through the actor. It is a play of mutual 'mirroring'. The audience supplies the communally constituted parts of the actor's body to the inspection of all. The actor is authorized by the audience, the audience by the actor. It is because the characters are fictional that we can push to the limits and involvements which we would not ordinarily dare to approach.
>
> (Wilshire 1982: 25)

Within this context we can explore all the possibilities of masks and unmasking and compare examples of authorization and absence thereof. If we think about the great theatrical characters, from the already quoted Oedipus to Antigone, from Hamlet to Richard III, from Nora (in Ibsen's *A Doll's House*) to Pirandello's *Six Characters*, to Beckett's bewildered existential clown (Vladimir and Estragon in *Waiting for Godot* or Hamm and Clov in *Endgame*), we realize that every one of them, in their own way, deals with the theme of authorization. We have already discussed Oedipus. Antigone, Oedipus's daughter (and therefore a participant in the myth), finds her fulfilment (as well as her end) in the conflict between an internal authority (pity, which is divine law) and an external one (the law of the *polis*). Hamlet problematically assumes the burden of the father figure who wants him to be an instrument of revenge against an illegitimate substitution by murder. It is to murder that Richard resorts to claim authorization that is denied to him because of his deformity. Nora fights to achieve the right of self-possession. In the last century, in which identity becomes more fragile, and paradoxically so, given the greater freedom from the conventions of social masks, the authority figure as a point of reference is missing. The struggle to find a source of authorization within ourselves, even though in conflict with recognized sources, is no longer possible. The 'Six Characters' go looking for an author to give them a reason for their existence. In much the same way the uprooted Vladimir and Estragon are confined to a timeless dimension, where they can do nothing but incessantly repeat the same patterns while waiting in vain for a utopian source of authorization. Hamm and Clov ape an attempt, through obsessive rituals, of mutual authorization to exist in a world that doesn't exist anymore.

The permission to explore

Exploration doesn't concern only the theme of authorization, which is reflected by the very nature of the basic principles of the theatre (the acceptance of the 'as if' paradox), but it can give rise to a virtually infinite range of potentialities of meaning. The character is located in the 'world' of drama by an actor who, like us, is a part of the world. It is at the centre of an endless network of projections and mimetic involvements, including both the spectator, who simultaneously participates in the world and the 'world', and the actor and their 'playmates':

> World and 'world' play into each other's hands, or there is no play at all. We cannot perceive the world in its own terms and then check to see if the terms of the 'world' reflect it accurately, for our sense of what the world is has already been determined in part from the play's 'world'. Nor, of course, can we decipher the 'world' of the play in terms that belong only to it, for its sense is an explication and development of the sense of the world.
>
> (Wilshire 1982: 40)

The theatrical character, therefore, lives in the intersecting area between world and 'world'. This area, which we will call *dramatic reality* (a concept which will be expanded upon later in this chapter), can be seen as *space/time of possibility*, which is both finite (because it is defined by a framework of rules, and indissolubly tied to elements of the world – the bodily reality of the actor) and infinite (because the limitations of space/time can be annulled, and because it reveals all the potentialities of meaning).

Performance/interpretation within the dramatic reality is in itself an act of transformation, for various reasons. First, because the legitimation of the Persona established by the dramatic action is itself temporary and subject to renegotiation. The mask can be changed at any moment, and it can even be taken off at the end of the performance (perhaps to be replaced by another, that of the actor in the world). In this sense, theatre gives an example of Persona's flexibility. What is more, the characters or Personae presented within the limitations of the 'world' are open to all possible mimetic connections, even those not immediately perceivable:

Take an actress playing Ophelia to an actor playing her father, Polonius. Granted, it is a fiction in certain fundamental ways; for example, the young woman enacting the older man's daughter is not necessarily his daughter offstage. We see this possibility as a part of seeing her enact the daughter onstage. As a contingent fact, she is not his daughter, but how about in essence? I use 'in essence' to refer to one's potentiality as a particular (say, sexed) member of the human species. Now, while the woman has no potentiality to be *this* man's daughter, she does have the potentiality to more deeply realize through acting with him, what the potentialities of being a daughter are; thus devolve upon her the potentiality of altering what she *is* as a daughter.

(Wilshire 1982: 104)

The actor who personifies the other mimetically internalizes all the aspects of the other relating to elements of his own individuality, and as the encounter is mediated by *performance/interpretation* within the 'as if' context, he has the possibility to consider these aspects from many points of view, including those that have never been approached in everyday life. By transforming the character, the actor transforms himself, and manifests this power in the presence of others.

Between 1989 and 1991, some of Shakespeare's plays were staged in the secure psychiatric hospital of Broadmoor, with the aim of provoking reactions that could activate therapeutic processes, an arduous task with this kind of patient. (On the meaning and results of the project see Cox 1982.) From the comments of the participants, it is clear that the emotional intensity of the performances was very high: after all, the audience was composed to a large extent of people who had committed crimes similar to those portrayed in *Hamlet* or *Measure for Measure*. Claire Higgins, an actress of the Royal Shakespeare Company, who played the role of Queen Gertrude, Hamlet's mother, comments on her encounter with the character of Ophelia:

Another mirror image – I see my silence reflected back by them (the two young people of the court who 'are cracking' as the play evolves), particularly Ophelia, whom I saw as an image of my younger self – forbidden to speak, controlled and manipulated by those around her. [. . .] When Ophelia breaks her silence through madness, I see my own choice: insanity or death.

(Cox 1982: 72)

The ambivalence (or shall we say polyvalence) of the comment is quite fascinating. We know that she is speaking on behalf of her character, but we realize that she is also talking about herself through Gertrude, and about herself in relation to Gertrude. But also about herself/Gertrude in relation to Ophelia, and to the actress playing Ophelia, to her and to the mirror of the audience. A spectator's testimony:

> This had me in tears because my sister who I love so much has been a victim of this most devastating crime of which I feel largely responsible.
>
> (Cox 1982:143)

Theatre makes possible the activation of a range of mimetic relationships (identification, projection, assumption and transfer), and by focusing them in a defined space/time, it makes them visible and comprehensible. The particular character, built through a multiplicity of relationships, makes the universal paradigms of relationships evident – and mimetically comprehensible. But at the same time, in virtue of its being *as if*, it shows the power of distance.

The theme of distance is what fully invests the figure of the actor. This topic merits particular attention, and will be further explored in the next section.

ACTOR AND CHARACTER

> Is it not monstrous that this player here,
> But in a fiction, in a dream of passion,
> Could force his soul so to his whole conceit
> That from her working all his visage wanned,
> Tears in his eyes, distraction in's aspect,
> A broken voice, and his whole function suiting
> With forms to his conceit? And all for nothing.
> For Hecuba!
> What's Hecuba to him, or he to Hecuba
> That he should weep for her?
>
> (Shakespeare, *Hamlet*)

Fictions

In the last period of his life, the Russian director Andrei Tarkovskij planned to make a film based upon Shakespeare's *Hamlet*, which he considered 'the greatest of all theatre works'. His untimely death deprived us of the greatest poetic director, and prevented the project's realization. In *Hamlet*, Tarkovskij saw 'the eternal problem of man being at a higher spiritual level, forced into contact with a lower and dirtier reality'. This interpretation reminds us of Tarkovskij's own drama, voluntarily exiled from his beloved country and in constant trouble in terms of funding his films (the latter fate was shared by other great directors such as Fellini and Kurosawa).

The unquestionable greatness of the most famous – and most staged – work of the Bard lies in its complexity and in the multiplicity of the meanings that can be assigned to it. For instance, the main theme of the substitution of the father, upon which we reflected in the preceding chapter, has opened the way to many philosophical and psychoanalytic interpretations. We are also deeply moved by other themes: those of doubt and indecision, of the struggles between life and death, of lost innocence, of the ambiguous bond between health and insanity. But the one which is perhaps most interesting for the purposes of this book is the theme of the relationship between theatre and life, a theme which is expressed in all of Shakespeare's works but particularly underlined and explicit in this play. It is underlined by the fact that is through dramatic action that the play comes to the revelation that can loosen the knots which support it. With *Mouse Trap*, made in what Victor Turner (1982) called the *subjunctive mode* (the 'as if' principle of dramatic action), Hamlet *captures the conscience of the king*, and forces him to reveal the deception and the crime that brought him to the throne (his father's illegitimate substitution and murder, which Hamlet cannot avenge but with another murder). It is made explicit in many illuminating statements on theatre scattered throughout the tragedy. At this point I would like briefly to consider the quotation at the beginning of this section, which Hamlet pronounces after having watched the actors' performance.

Hamlet states that the actor, 'but in a fiction, in a dream of passion, could force his soul so to his whole conceit' in such a way that he and the spectators watching him experience the effects of amazing metamorphoses. He asks how it is possible: 'What's Hecuba to him, or he to Hecuba?'

We can suppose that, for Hamlet, the issue of playing a part (to take on a Persona) is a particularly meaningful one, considering that during the play he must, at times against his will, play many of them: the roles of the devoted son and subject, the lover, the friend, the wise man and the madman, the astute person and the dull one, the innocent party and the guilty one. And all this happens *in a fiction*. It must be said that the

Italian translation cannot render the complete sense of the term fiction. The Italian verb *fingere* has the primary meaning 'to make someone believe what is not true, to simulate'. Thus, it contains the theme of deception in its semantic range (the deception of the actor we considered before). In the English term 'fiction', this element is rather slight, the major meaning being related to the action of telling. Fiction designates the presence of a narrative framework, not necessarily aimed at simulate Reality; on the contrary its nature is openly declared. When Hamlet affirms that the actor is 'in a fiction', he is saying that the action moves within a narrative dimension, evoked by the actor himself and shared by the spectator, which doesn't pretend to be reality (at least not everyday reality as it is conventionally agreed), but that nevertheless possesses some particular characteristics of credibility and shareability. On the other hand, the Latin verb *fingo* refers in its primary meaning to the art of the potter and the sculptor, who give form to raw material with their own hands: 'to form, to shape, to mould, to carve' (bringing to mind the biblical God who created man from dust). In a figurative sense it means (besides 'to pretend, to simulate') 'to make, to create', and also 'to form, to educate, to instruct', and finally 'to imagine, to fancy, to suppose'.

> Sempre caro mi fu quest'ermo colle,
> E questa siepe, che da tanta parte
> Dell'ultimo orizzonte il guardo esclude.
> Ma sedendo e mirando, interminati
> Spazi di là da quella, e sovrumani
> Silenzi, e profondissima quiete
> Io nel pensier mi fingo . . .
> (Giacomo Leopardi, *L'infinito*, 1831)

* *

> Always dear to me was this remote hill,
> And this hedge, that from so many places
> Along the distant horizon excludes the eye.
> But sitting and contemplating, endless
> Spaces beyond there, and superhuman
> Silences and deep quiet
> I pretend in my thoughts . . .

The existential importance of this *pretence* is underlined by the fact that, even if the likelihood of finding a garbage dump or an unauthorized building behind that hedge is much greater today than in Leopardi's time, these lines still move us. The act of pretending is first and foremost a creative act.

To continue our discussion of *Hamlet*, the condition in which this narrative dimension is generated is that of a *dream of passion*. Is it the dreamed emotion or the dream that becomes emotion? Whatever the answer may be, we are talking about something that does not easily submit to the control of will and intentions (of the consciousness). Whatever their source, be it supernatural or the deep recesses of our psyche, dreams are always something that we cannot intentionally govern. According to psychoanalysis, the school of thought that has focused perhaps more than any other on dreams, they develop along clear lines, similar to a theatre show. Fausto Petrella, one of the most eminent Italian psychoanalysts, has written:

> If we examine how Freud conceives the constructive principles of the dream, we see that they are entirely comparable to scenic operations and to the actors' stage calls, which share different parts. What he calls *oneiric work* resembles the work required for staging a dramatic sequence, but starting from a text that originally was not destined to theatre. A text that, in the case of the dreamer, is unknown to himself and must be deducted by stage enactments.
>
> (Petrella 1985: 41)

The possibility for the dreamer to be an active part in creating and directing the dream is a recurring desire in the history of mankind. The connections between the conscious self and the dream remain mysterious and fascinating.

On the other hand, *passion* refers to the fact that feelings cannot be governed when they are interwoven with instinctual drives. The etymology of the word passion includes the idea of suffering. Daniel Goleman, in his documented study on *emotional intelligence*, describes the phenomenon of *emotional sequestration*, the domination of the whole personality by archaic areas of the brain (the amygdala and the hippocampus), to the detriment of more evolved parts (the new cortex, which is responsible for language acquisition and rational thought).

The *dream of passion* starting inside a fictional framework can therefore seem very similar to possession. The mask penetrates deep into the actor and pervades their whole personality. But, on a more basic level, the process that makes all of this possible is of a deliberate and rational kind. The actor *forces his soul to his whole conceit*, consciously imposing the other on himself or rather (as previously discussed), on what he considers to be himself – provisionally and in a certain sense arbitrarily. Indeed, the monstrosity and the wonder of the actor's art lie in this paradox, in which the reality/fiction dichotomy is annulled and the action takes place on the thresholds of possible worlds, each of which being a reality level, which can be crossed at will.

The actor's paradox

Theatrical thought in the last centuries has focused on the actor's paradox, defined by Robert Landy in a reversal of Hamlet's doubt as 'To be *and* not to be'. When Denis Diderot expresses this paradox in his famous lines from *Paradoxe sur le comédien*, he provides a compelling solution to it. It is only a matter of pretence, in the sense of an honest deception:

> That cracking of the voice, those uncertain words, those smothered or prolonged sounds, that quivering of the limbs, that staggering of the knees, those faints and those impetuses: pure imagination, lessons prepared in advance, pathetic grimaces, sublime aping, preserved for a long time in the actor's memory, after having studied, of which he lacks a precise awareness in the moment of the performance, and that allows him, fortunately for the poet, the spectator and himself, to keep his mind totally free, requiring only, as every other exercise, physical strength.
>
> (Diderot 1830: 81)

According to Diderot, it is the total absence of sensibility that makes an actor great. His consciousness, in assuming a Persona, demonstrates total control of the body-self, which allows him to show all the effects of the feelings without being affected by them in any way:

> The tears of the true actor are shed by the brain; those of the sensitive man by the heart. In the sensitive man the bowels excessively upset the head; in the actor it is the head that sometimes causes a momentary disturbance in the bowels.
>
> (Diderot 1830: 82)

The amygdala has nothing to do with all this. The action of the actor is a mimesis without involvement. Diderot doesn't exclude the possibility of emotional involvement, but it happens only sometimes and it is in any event a momentary disturbance.

The man who took this idea of separation (absolute distance) to an extreme, to the point of creating an ideology based upon it, was Bertolt Brecht. His concept of *estrangement* has the function of setting off a cognitive awareness both in the actor and the audience, aimed at raising political awareness, and therefore stimulating collective action. Emotional involvement can indeed inhibit the action (one can be frozen by emotion, as, for instance, with fear), or can start out uncontrolled and potentially destructive acting (Goleman's *emotional sequestration*). Being a Marxist, Brecht longed for a transformation of the world based on reason. The actor must therefore reflect on the character and expose it objectively, without denying any emotional implications but rather experiencing them while remaining detached from them:

> Certainly, everything she did made her seem to be
> A fisherman's woman; she also did not
> Identify herself with that woman totally,
> But she acted as if
> Another thought filled her mind
> And she asked herself: but what was she like?
> Even if you could not always guess
> What she thought about that character, you understood all the same
> That she was thinking about it, and that she invited
> Others to think about it.
>   (Bertolt Brecht, *Description of the way of acting of H.W.*)

Brecht puts the issue of distance at the extreme polarity of separation, introducing the necessity of a person/Persona relationship in acting that includes observation. I can observe myself acting in virtue of the fact that the action doesn't involve me.

In the Indian *Bhagavad Gita*, the god Krishna, disguised as a charioteer, provides answers to Arjuna's doubts about taking action or not (in a way the same doubts expressed by Hamlet with his 'To be or not to be'): whether to begin a devastating battle against his own kinsmen or to surrender and be destroyed. The god orders Arjuna to take action, but to eliminate any passion from his actions:

> Be involved only in the action, never being interested with the fruits. [...] Complete your actions, Arjuna, being so firm in the yoga, having abandoned the attachment. Be equal in the success and in the failure. [...] The one whose deeds are, without exception, devoid of

desire's bond, he who offers everything to the renunciation, this is a
true wise man!

(*Bhagavad Gita*, II: 49)

The attitude of the wise man must be like that of the god, who contem-
plates his own actions with the detached eye of the spectator:

These actions, Arjuna, are not for me source of any bond, because,
as the indifferent one, I assist to these actions, detached.

(ibid. IX: 10)

The suppression of feeling makes the action pure and effective in a story
(the *Mahābhārata*, the immense epic poem which contains the *Bhagavad
Gita*), characterized by deep and destructive passions. In the end this
detached action provokes the total destruction of mankind, from which a
new one will arise.

Peter Brook, who has directed a memorable play based on the
Mahābhārata, deals with this philosophical and psychological dilemma
(observing ourselves in the heat of action) in theatrical terms, by
indicating yet another paradox:

Because the great mystery is that the more the actor gets involved,
and, if he's a good actor, the more he gives body and soul to the
enactment, the more he is, at the same time, internally free; his
internal distance increases with the commitment, which is a paradox.
The same thing happens to the audience. A really interested audience
is at the same time free to look with a certain objectivity what they
are intensely living in a subjective way.

(Di Bernardi 1989: 148–9)

From paradox to paradox, we are thus getting to the very heart of the
matter expressed by Hamlet's reflection, that is in itself a paradox, in
the sense that it requires the acceptance of two opposing truths: that the
actor is entirely *himself* and *the other*, feeling the feelings of the other while
preserving his own; that he wholly participates at the same time in the
world and in the 'world'. To consider these two truths as complementary
rather than incompatible calls for an intense imaginative effort; and it
leaves the question of *how* unresolved – the greatest mystery which Brook
speaks about. What process is set off between the actor and character,
allowing this paradoxical synthesis between *being* and *appearing*?

So near, so far

Having quoted Brecht, we have to take into account an author who, rightly or wrongly, is commonly considered to be the representative of the opposite polarity in the conception of the actor–character relationship: Kostantin Stanislavskij. Unlike Brecht, who was above all a writer and a director with a penchant for theatre's pedagogic and political mission, Stanislavskij had been himself an actor for many years. As an actor, he could not accept the idea of an acting without sensitivity as suggested by Diderot (who, we must remember, never trod the stage); a purely mental mimesis, in which the living body is degraded from a living centre of feelings and emotions to a mere technical tool. Stanislavskij's research springs from his personal dissatisfaction with that kind of theatrical formality, and comes to what is now universally known (thanks to his American followers, who greatly influenced Hollywood) as The Method; even if it may sound odd that what can be seen as an attempt to reintroduce the actor's emotional world in his art is defined by a term fully belonging to 'pure' scientific thought. Stanislavskij develops a procedure for approaching the character that follows an imaginative path. The *ifs* and the *given circumstances*, which are the premises of this process, require the actor to use his imagination, allowing him to approach the *Other* through an amplification of his own feelings that leads to a process of universalization. However, Stanislavskij warns that 'the actor, once on stage, always remains himself, and he acts in the first person'.

The universal feelings of the character are expressed from within the actor, not as abstract concepts but in virtue of belonging to the range of possibilities, connecting the human world to the world of fiction. This encounter between actor and character (which is neither a fusion nor a pretence) includes an emotional level. But it doesn't deal with raw, immediate emotion, the reaction to the event here and now: the *emotional memory* that Stanislavskij places at the centre of the actor's work is the filtered emotion, matured with time, evoked by the imaginative encounter. It is the opposite of what happens to us each day, when emotions invade us and only later are recognized and named (the activation of the limbic system, then the intervention of the new cortex, see Goleman 1995). Without a doubt, this flow of imagination/emotion through the fiction (the narrative frame) is the same type of process that happens in the theatre audience, and the audience of any narration in general. The wolf of *Little Red Riding Hood* evokes but also contains the child's sense of fear. But if I tell the story filling it too much with my own fear, the emotion will be too unbalanced in the *here and now* to allow the child to benefit from it. A communion must take place between narrator and listener (between actor and spectator), what Martin Buber called 'the sphere of the inter-human', of the subject/subject relationship.[1]

If we consider this necessity in terms of the actor/character relationship, that is, of the encounter with the imagined other, we see that the process is again one of mutual influencing. The synthesis of performance/interpretation happens through a transformation both of the actor and of the character. Even when the character is tied to the text, its actualization on stage is a unique meeting. You cannot give two identical performances of the same character. As Georg Simmel noticed in one of his illuminating essays on the philosophy of the actor:

> There is not only, on the one hand, the objective task fixed by the writer and, on the other, the concrete subjectivity of the actor, so that it would be enough for the latter to conform himself to the former. Instead, a third aspect must be added to these two: the demands that the role makes upon this actor and perhaps no other; the particular law that derives from this role for this actor's personality.
>
> (Simmel 1908: 29)

In the space between the actor and the character an imaginative tide comes to life, which separates and connects, permitting the passage of emotions, yet being under the control of the consciousness. This space is similarly present in the relationship between spectator and actor: the setting in motion of a flow of mimetic identifications and, at the same time, a position of separation and objectiveness. The audience neverthe-less comes into contact with the actor as character (which underlines, through the description of a particular person, a *type* of person, or at least a visible segment of the behaviour of a potential person, on which the spectator can project parts of himself), but also as a person who, partici-pating in the common human condition of being a physical body, realizes the potentiality of mimetic flows:

> Stated analytically, the actor in the world stands in for the character in the 'world', and thereby stands in also for us – we who are likewise in the world. Speaking experientially, however, we must say that the body of the actor speaks directly to us, and for us.
>
> (Wilshire 1982: 40)

In the same way, we can locate this imaginative space/flow in the relation-ship between the *Text*, the *performing actor* and the *interpreting actor*.

With *Text* we mean the pre-existing forms, in which we include the Personae and the culturally and traditionally determined behaviours, but also those archetypal figures that, according to Jung, dwell in the collective soul. The *performing actor* puts into action his personal version of the pre-existing forms. The *interpreting actor* composes meanings, observes and judges. In everyday life, this triangular relationship is only partially governed by the consciousness. In drama, the narrative dimension (as if) makes it possible to regulate the mimetic flows and to extend or reduce the distance.

But let's try to examine in detail this approaching path between the actor and the character as Stanislavskij has conceived it:

> I try asking myself a more difficult question, that is, what was Cackij feeling while he was going to Famusov and to Sofia? I start noticing a feeling of uneasiness come over me, as if I am losing my balance, and I am afraid of a constraint. How can I guess another's feelings, how can I put myself in his shoes, how can I take his place? I quickly reformulate the question: 'What do people who are in love do when, as in the case of Cackij, they return to their beloved after years of separation? Put this way, the question appears less scary to me, but arid, vague and generic, and I am quick to reformulate it differently: 'What would I do now if I were going, not to the theatre, but to my 'woman', it doesn't matter which, Sofia or Natasha?
>
> (Stanislavskij 1963: 55)

The conscious 'I' undergoes a construction process that allows him to compare himself to the Other, but this comparison can result in a loss of equilibrium, a mimetic engulfment that annuls the chance for the individual to be free and to be the master of himself. This can be frightening: it is, in fact, an illegitimate substitution, a *becoming the Other* involving a loss of identity. The possibility for this encounter to occur implies a shift from the particular to the universal: the manifestation of a potentially shareable way of being, as an expression of the manifold, even if not endless, variations on human existence. This shift opens another possibility: to participate in, or more precisely *through*, the epiphany of the Other, while preserving our own individuality. Quoting Simmel again:

> The pre-existing form of theatrical art consists in the fact that the human being lives or performs as if a pre-existing 'Other' were his own autonomous development. He, however, doesn't simply abandon

his own being but fills with it the other, and divides the flow of this 'Other' in manifold rivulets, each of which, also flowing into a preliminarily given river bed, contains the whole inner being in a particular structure.

(Simmel 1920/21: 55)

We can return at this point to Hamlet's crucial question, and attempt to provide our own personal answer. Hecuba flows in these manifold rivulets, and every one of them has a potentially shareable existential meaning: wife, mother, victim and avenger, custodian and evoker of innumerable other roles, embryonic or potential, that belong to me as a human creature. And I am for Hecuba that unique, precious place where their incarnation is possible.

DRAMATIC REALITY

Who did she meet, then?
Well, she didn't meet anybody for a long time. But after a while this little girl named I sees another little girl just like her.
You mean this other little girl looked like this little girl named I?
Just just just like her.
That was funny, wasn't it?
Yes, it was. And I said to this other little girl: 'What's your name?' I said 'Because I'd like to know' and this other little girl she never said anything.
Not anything?
No. And then I said to this other little girl, just like this I said: 'Who are you?'
And what did this other little girl say?
'You. That's who I am,' she said. 'And You is my name because I'm You.'
I suppose this little girl named I was surprised?
I was ever so surprised.
And what happened then?
Then I said to You, 'Would you like to have some tea?' I said. And You said 'Yes. I would' You said.

(E.E. Cummings, *The Little Girl Named I*, 1965)

Threshold as a physical place

The stage, the place where the dramatic action is brought to life, is first a physical location, and therefore we must think of it as being endowed with those qualities we usually ascribe to the physical world: extension in space and permanence in time. Dramatic space/time requires established boundaries, which separate it from the background, expressed by signs that one can understand and share. Precisely because the theatre doesn't simulate reality but creates a new one, it is always necessary to allow comparison to be made, and the spatial signs make it possible to visualize the lines of separation along which this comparison (which is an encounter as well) can happen. These signs can be extremely evident, made of stone or wood, or can even be extremely subtle: a circle formed by people's bodies. They are in any case intelligible; they are the interfaces that separate and connect the world and the 'world'. The space/time dimension of the stage is a threshold.

> Threshold: what is for two lovers
> To wear out a little
> The ancient threshold of their own house,
> Even them, after the many in the past,
> And before those who will come . . . lightly.
> (Rainer Maria Rilke, *Duineser Elegies*, *X*, 1923)

Rilke's image evokes the act of crossing the home threshold by the newly married bride and groom, a central part of the nuptial rite in ancient Rome (see Bianconi 1999). After some ritualized phrases were pronounced, the threshold was greased with wolf fat, and the bride was carried across it in the bridegroom's arms, so that her feet didn't touch the ground. In this ritual passage, the crossing of the threshold enacts a transformation: a change of status in the social universe and a change of meaning in the symbolic universe. Nevertheless, the image also reminds us of the moment of *time without time* that is created between two lovers just before their temporary separation; the threshold is worn out under their feet, testifying the presence of physical bodies, but *lightly*, as though to tell us that the state of fusion preceding the separation, which is, in a certain sense, part of it, has a slightly different quality of existence. It is time without time, as we have said, in the sense of an internal perception of the passing of time, not synchronized with the movement of the clock; the moment of eternity within the limitations of 'before' and 'after', of 'inside' and 'outside'. It is the 'world in a grain of sand and the sky in a wild flower' that

Holds Infinity in the palm of a hand,
Eternity in an hour.
(William Blake, *Auguries of Innocence*)

Can we think of a definite place in space and time within which space and time are recreated, manifesting themselves in a different way? From a Kantian point of view, we must assume that space and time are not inherent to things in themselves, but to our ability to know them (or rather to sense them). On the threshold, space cannot be measured geometrically, and time cannot be divided arithmetically. In other words, the individual and collective experience of the threshold's space/time can be qualitatively different from the experience of everyday space/time, but it is nonetheless a lived experience (an *Erlebnis*, according to Dilthey). Therefore it exerts a fundamental influence in the person's constructing processes shared by the human community.

The journey inside the threshold

This phenomenon is particularly evident in rites. A rite is an organized set of actions and events, situated in a fixed space and time. But inside it, the region of the myth is extended. The myth is a network of religious symbols referring to a level of experience that goes beyond sensory experience, of which, according to Kant, space and time are a priori forms of intuition. In the collective ritual, the symbolic epiphany inside the community occurs in the narrative configuration of the myth, which can be expressed both through narration (as a text) and through form (as a subtext or implicit text). An example of the first type is the *Hako* ritual of the Pawnee Indians, as described by Alice Fletcher (1904). In this ritual the story of the Mother of Wheat and her search for the Son is told in detail with songs, objects and dramatic actions. The whole community takes part in the performance, renewing the power of generation and nourishment. On the contrary, in the Mysteries of Eleusis the myth is a frame of reference exposed through signs/symbols shown to the initiate: the stalk of wheat, the basket/womb, the fire. In a similar fashion, the bread and wine of the Catholic mass are incorporated by the person who receives communion, thus participating in the story of Christ's death and resurrection.

> Throughout the world, in corporate rituals, men and women perform symbolic journeys, back to the source of the life, yet knowing their journey to be a passage, forward to a richer life, a more secure place than where we are
>
> (Grainger 2000: 3)

The symbolic journey is a journey in the threshold's space/time dimension. It is nonetheless a journey, which preserves some fundamental structures and meanings of the journey in its purer form (archetypal, one could say). There is a preparation stage, in which one takes into consideration the itinerary, with its foreseeable elements and its inevitable aspects of mystery and the unexpected. One must pack one's bags and prepare oneself to face the fatigue of the journey and possible encounters with the unknown. The central part is the journey itself, which involves leaving familiar places and habits behind and encountering new things (people, landscapes, modes of expression, events) that can cause anxiety and are potentially dangerous, yet challenging. We risk losing our identity, but if we succeed in finding the proper balance to face them, these things can lead to renewed knowledge and a new harmony within ourselves. The third stage is that of the return, in which the changes that have taken place inside us enter into relationship with the world that we have temporarily abandoned, thereby modifying it.

Of course, this kind of journey is not like today's organized trips, in which everything is prepared in detail, unforeseen events are considered bothersome and the desire for the unusual is relegated to a voyeur dimension. It is perhaps more similar to the 'hero's journey', defined as the 'mono-myth' by Joseph Campbell (1949), which is present in all ages and cultures in dreams and fairy tales. Robert Landy, defining the figure of the hero in his *Taxonomy of Roles*, writes:

> The hero journeys forth on a spiritual search that proves in some way to be transformational. [The hero] is moral, inquisitive, and open to confronting the unknown. The classical heroes are those who search for a meaning just beyond their grasp, willing to confront the hardship of the journey and to accept the tragic consequences that arise from uncovering certain elemental ambivalences of being. [. . .] Thus, the function of the hero is to take a risky spiritual and psychological journey toward understanding and transformation.
>
> (Landy 1993: 230)

As if

This quest for knowledge within the threshold's borders can be under-taken, in rite as in drama, in virtue of that kind of relationship between the individual and the world that we have defined 'as if', involving an act of will (and therefore of the consciousness) in the 'suspension of disbelief' and in the acceptance of a hypothesis of reality as a constructive possibility. The process of identification/separation between actor and character, as we have seen, can start with a deliberate action of 'as if', as well as the process of identification/separation between spectator and actor/character. However, Grainger reminds us:

> As *if* signifies more than 'pretending to be someone else', or even 'imagining something or someone to be different from how I first perceived them.' In fact, it denotes a principle basic to humanness itself: that of freedom or flexibility of thought, and therefore of experience.
>
> (Grainger and Duggan 1997: 2)

We could affirm that this basic principle is the same one with which our very personality is formed, since the first primary process of identification/separation (mimetic merging/differentiation). Winnicott dedicates some memorable reflections to the *transitional object* that the child uses as an intermediary between himself and his mother to overcome in a non-destructive way the difficulties arising from the first imperfections in the original mimetic fusion. The child's use of transitional objects cannot be ascribed, except in a metaphorical sense, to an act of will, unless we understand the term *will* not as a conscious intention of the self, but rather as Schopenhauer intended: as a fundamental principle of the world in itself, which becomes objective in our body-self (our individuality).

> This intermediate area of experience, regardless of whether it belongs to internal or external (shared) reality, forms the greatest part of the child's experience, and it is preserved throughout his entire life in intense experiences that belong to the arts, to religion, to an imaginative way of life and creative work in general.
>
> (Winnicott 1971: 43)

The transitional object is not a sort of artifice contrived by the child to bear the pain of separation, but the application in a specific context of a potentiality inscribed in human nature, which is closely linked to creativity. Comments Grainger: 'A child's first important toy is his or her first work of art' (2000: 2).

Similarly, we could say that art as a whole is a transitional phenomenon, a threshold phenomenon. The work of art expresses the internal world of its creator, but it is placed as an object in the external world. It is precisely its visible nature that facilitates separation and therefore the relationship between two worlds. When the imaginative world and the external world merge, becoming indistinguishable, the individual is faced with a fleeting and unpredictable reality, in which the categories that we normally use for anticipating events (what Kelly 1963 calls *personal constructs*) are no longer applicable, or even never existed in a permanent way. A world like this can be frightening. This condition, which Silvano Arieti calls *a-dualism*, is typical of the delirium characterizing the most serious forms of schizophrenia. But the work of art, continues Arieti:

> belongs to a second reality, which maintains a certain distance from the first reality. It differs from the delirious 'reality' of the psychotic person, which is fused with the first reality and therefore belongs to it. In the creative action the artist sees his work of art as independent from him and already endowed with its own life. [. . .] Art's a-dualism turns into *aesthetic distance*.
>
> (Arieti 1976: 197)

Unlike other threshold phenomena such as dreams, trances and deliria, the potentiality of the boundaries' definition is maintained in art and can be thematized: it is thus both cognitive in the strict sense and intuitively experienced. Artistic processes, and particularly dramatic processes, are based on the balance between flow and control, between intuition and language.

A child is able to play, and to do so intentionally, a long time before being able to conceive the 'play' category in conceptual terms (and a long time before being able to verbally communicate the meta-message 'this is play'). Actually, playing is not an activity but a 'framework of events' (see Bateson 1979), whose boundaries are outlined to a great extent by non-verbal messages. These mimetic messages are related to the body (posture, tension, equilibrium and many other body signals) and can be observed in children and young mammals at play. Anyone who has ever dealt with a puppy knows that the invitation to play, from both parties, is difficult to describe in terms of a sequence of actions; nevertheless it is unequivocal. The pup and his playmate create a shared dimension together, in which relational events take on special meaning, distinct from their meaning in other areas of experience located out of the play frame: in it, a bite does not harm. When the play becomes more complex, and the fictional dimension enters into its structure, the relationship between the world of play and the world of non-play develops into a network of mutual references. It is necessary that the borders be declared in advance and comprehensible. The meta-message that 'this is play', whether verbalized or not, has to be explicitly expressed. On the other hand, if we consider the famous opening line of Peter Brook's book (quoted before), we have to admit that the first action on which the theatre is based is an attribution of sense (a linguistic act): 'I can take an empty space and call it bare scene'. Once the borders are clarified, the dramatic contract (the acceptance of *as if*) is implicit in the dramatic act itself, both from the actor's and the spectator's point of view. Shakespeare has the choir of Henry V pronounce the following words:

> Can this cock-pit hold
> The vasty fields of France? Or may we cram
> Within this wooden O the very casques
> That did affright the air at Agincourt?
> O pardon: since a crookèd figure may
> Attest in little place a million,
> And let us, ciphers to this great account,
> On your imaginary forces work.
>
> *(Henry V*, Prol.)

Imagination

The *imaginary forces* to which Shakespeare makes an appeal as a condition for the dramatic event to take place, is the faculty that allows the creation of a *middle course* between the external/internal world, control/flux and intuition/language polarities. To clarify this, I would start considering a definition of the imagination provided not by a poet but by a psychiatrist. According to Arieti:

> Imagination is the ability of the mind to produce or to reproduce many symbolic functions in a conscious, wakeful state, without any voluntary effort to reproduce such functions.
>
> (Arieti 1976: 41)

Therefore, to imagine is not simply to reproduce (internally or externally) what is absent in some or all of its visible aspects. The iconic imagination (what Arieti calls *Imaginative*) is an essential element in the imagination process, but it is not the only one. The symbolic functions of which Arieti speaks concern the complexity of the individual, even in an emotional sense; not only because 'the image allows a human being to preserve an emotional attitude toward an absent object' (Stanislavskij's emotional memory), but also because the symbols are twofold objects, portraying both the visible and the invisible, reality and possibility. The symbolic functions open the channels of communication between the individual and the world, in a relational process of understanding the world that develops along the interpretation/performance axis. Imagination is related to the ability to produce symbols, therefore to language and communication, and it is always accompanied by a certain affective quality that legitimizes it as a lived experience. If the imaginative process (beginning with the transitional object) is not available, not only the world of artistic creativity is denied, but also the possibility to interact with the world in creative ways, in a flow of mutual transformation.

Arieti shows how the imaginative process, once activated, develops somehow autonomously, escaping deliberate attempts to control it: it can slip from our fingers and overcome us. In the mental condition that psychiatrists call *paranoia*, defined by the DSM IV as 'a pervasive distrust and suspiciousness of others so that their intentions are interpreted as malevolent', the imagination becomes fixed on recurrent constructions bearing strong emotional connotations that make it impermeable to comparisons with the other reality, the shared reality of the everyday world, banal but necessary for survival. In Gombrowicz's novel *Cosmos*, the protagonist is constantly seeing threatening signs in the minute details of his surrounding environment, signs that are related to each other, thus creating the condition of anxious anticipation of an imminent catastrophe:

> How could we pretend not to notice: the hanged sparrow – the hanging cane – the cane hung up on the wall which brought to mind the bird hanging from the bush – a strange effect that subsequently increased the intensity of the sparrow. It was difficult not to think that someone had led us to the cane, to connect it to the sparrow . . . but why? For what purpose? A joke? A prank? Someone was making fun of us, jeering at us, having a good laugh at our expense.
>
> (Gombrowicz 1965)

Reality is transformed by the imagination locked behind the heavy bars of a jail: the whole world seems to be plotting against us and manifests this fact with signs that we are forced to interpret. The process of interpretation/performance, in the presence of a blocked imagination, becomes repetitive and leads down blind alleys. Writes the psychiatrist Giovanni Jervis:

> According to a description dating from psychiatric research of the last century, a semi-delirious experience of persecution can be brought

on voluntarily by an exercise: it is enough to go out walking in a less familiar neighbourhood, and while walking, to try to convince ourselves that everybody is looking at us and making conventional signs. Such an exercise, if done well, gives rise in a short time in the majority of people who try it to the very painful feeling of not being able to free oneself from the hostile and secret attention of others.

(Jervis 1975: 247)

A simple imaginative exercise can produce such great effects, even at a physical level (the somatic outcome of emotion): the *power of imagination* spreads to the power of possession. It is somewhat similar to the actor of whom Hamlet speaks: 'all his visage waned, Tears in his eyes, distraction in's aspect'. But the actor has an extra resource. He governs his own imagination. He leads it and lets it lead him down new paths without losing his way back. The actor's imagination is *poetic imagination* in the etymological sense of the word *poiesis*, meaning to call into existence something that can be perceived as different from what already exists, producing new knowledge. This kind of imagination is not idiosyncratic fantasy, withdrawn into the self and incommunicable: rather, it is generation of meaning, therefore a creative power directed toward the world.

William Blake,[2] following Paracelsus, distinguished Fantasy, the mere daydream, similar to illusion, deception and self-deception, from Imagination, the supreme human faculty. A few months before his death, Blake wrote to his friend Cumberland:

I have been very near the Gates of Death and have returned very weak & an Old Man feeble and tottering, but not in Spirit & Life not in The Real Man The Imagination which Liveth for Ever.

We can see how, in Blake's view, Imagination is not only a central element of human experience, but also the fundamental possibility of connecting the parts of the world, including ourselves within it, through the vital gesture of conferring sense. Milton O. Percival has written:

[According to Blake], from Imagination comes that identification of one self with another which insures brotherhood and the forgiveness of sin. From Imagination, with its capacity to accept every minute particular of life, taking home to one's bosom a share of responsibility for particulars which self-righteousness would condemn, comes the perfect unity which is beyond rational achievement or even rational conception. From Imagination comes the conception of life as ever changing, ever expanding, and the consequent release of energy for imaginative ends, which is the prime source of Blakean delight.

(Percival 1937: 50)

In Blake's masterpiece, the poem *Jerusalem*, the giant Albion, symbol of humanity but also of England, of the individual in their psychic complexity and of the poet himself, lies sleeping. While asleep, his soul breaks apart, giving birth to four different creatures: Urthona, Intuition; Tharmas, Body; Luvah, Feeling; Urizen, Reason. The disjunction produces chaos, war and a general loss of sense, underlined by the exile of Albion's female counterpart: Jerusalem, incarnation of Liberty. Singing, the poet Los (Urthona's son) sets his Spectre (the rational power of the divided man) to work: he will stoke the fire in the Furnaces of Affliction, through which the alchemical work of transformation will be completed, up to the conclusive synthesis in the *conjunctio oppositorum*.

Los's tools are song and fire, but his energy comes from the Imagination. S. Foster Damon (1965) writes of Blake, 'Imagination is the central faculty of both God and man; indeed, here the two become indistinguishable.'

All Things Exist in the Human Imagination [. . .]
In your own Bosom you bear your Heaven and Earth & all
you behold, Tho' it appears Without, is Within.

(Blake, *Jerusalem*)

Imagination is the central element of the creative action, the complete freedom of the spirit, which connects us with a superior reality (Huxley's Divine Reality) but it relates to the world through form.

Nature has no Outline, but Imagination has. Nature has no Tune, but Imagination has. Nature has no Supernatural & dissolves: Imagination is Eternity.

(*The Ghost of Abel*)

In the vision of Jerusalem, imagination connects the different elements of human experience, not attempting to deny the tensions and the conflicts among them, but transfiguring them in a higher vision.[3] In a certain sense, it plays the same role as Jung's *Transcendent Function*: 'the dynamic event through which all the psychic elements (which both in practical and cognitive-affective terms had been previously distinguished and were labelled by then as contrary or extraneous) are reassembled in a non synthetic unity, neither intellectualistic nor aesthetic, even though they need an intellectual and aesthetic representation' (Pieri 1998: 300). The power of the imagination that brings the teddybear to life and populates a circular stage with helmets and spears allows us to build sketches of the world, made visible through the creative process. At the same time, it allows us temporarily to abandon ourselves in search of otherness. Writes Grainger:

> Imagination is really another dimension of personal and social being, one which whenever I enter it releases me from my preoccupation with my own actions and intentions and sets me free to pursue the completeness I long for and do not find anywhere except in encountering the otherness which establishes my own very separate personal identity. This is a doctrine of the imagination which allows it to perform a completely different role from that of an expression of the self – that of moving beyond itself to find a new way of being itself.
>
> (Grainger and Duggan 1997: 18)

The other: risk and safety

Although it is an individual journey, the imaginative journey within the threshold is not accomplished alone, but with other human beings. People make their awareness of the shared human condition available to others, with its weakness and vulnerability, but also with the evocation and discovery of its power, the power to transform others as well as ourselves. This power is the recognition of what humanistic psychologists have called the *human potential*, intending the presence in everyone of 'an underground flow of movement toward a constructive realization of our inherent possibilities, a natural tendency toward a more complex and complete development' (Rogers 1961). In other terms, this idea suggests that in human beings the process that Maturana and Varela (1980) have defined *auto-poiesis* (the ability of organisms as complex systems to build and to reorganize themselves by elaborating the stimuli of the environment in structural terms) must be reinterpreted in teleological terms. Or perhaps it would be more exact to say *teleonomic*, following Lorenz's specifications (1983), who insists on the fact that we can attribute the sense of an Aristotelian *final cause* (which, among the dynamic causes, is the opposite of the *efficient cause*, the latter being a 'coming from', rather than a 'going to') to the transformation of living systems. But even by applying this concept to the transformation of living things, we can suppose that it has some purpose, but we do not know what. In our understanding of human beings (and in our effort to build an explanatory model of it), this idea translates as an act of faith in human nature, comparable to an act of poetic faith, in recognizing the search for happiness, for wholeness, and for self-realization as particular characteristics of human nature.

On the basis of the reflections we have made upon the relational making of individuality, we may hypothesize that these human characteristics can be developed through mimetic relationships. However, they can also be trapped or inhibited by them.

Dramatic reality, which possesses a 'transitional' quality founded upon 'as if', is the physical and mental place where mimetic relationships can be enacted without irreversible consequences for the life of the person. Within this space it is possible to check the distance between oneself and the other and to observe oneself in the heat of the action; to be a vehicle of unknown powers, while maintaining one's own identity; to experience Personae and masks without having to keep them for the rest of one's life; to open the gates of emotion with the security that they can be closed once again.

> In the shared world of the imagination, 'as if' achieves epistemological value as a way of approaching human truth.
>
> (Grainger 1999: 22)

The purpose of this 'journey within the threshold' is not historically to retrace the mimetic/relational patterns of each individual, seen as efficient causes of their discomfort and unhappiness now, but to allow everyone to rediscover the potentiality of being in the flow of life, remaining all the while in control of it – the 'flexibility and liberty of thought and experience' of which Grainger speaks; in other words, the constructive and creative side of the person/world relationship, which influences the balance between being adjusted to reality and transforming it, allowing us to see ourselves as the authors of our own destiny and the heroes of our own quest for knowledge. The relationship between body, consciousness and appearance can be re-enacted inside the protective framework of 'as if', allowing endless possibilities of recomposition: the same possibilities offered by life that we are not always able to take advantage of, set as we are in our position of withdrawal or defence/attack with respect to the world. But in the 'as if' dimension the possibilities are assembled in the universe of dramatic reality, and the artistic essence of the individual or collective production process of this reality makes it present and lived, visible and shareable. I agree with Wilshire when he writes:

> Theatre is a mode of discovery that explores the threads of what is implicit and buried in the world, pulls them into a compressed and acknowledgeable pattern before us in its 'world'.
>
> (1982: xiv)

What is more, the fact that this journey is undertaken in the company of others implies a mutual authorization, a mutual concession of the 'permission to exist'.

Of course, the group can also represent an obstacle, becoming a screen on which one projects one's 'unfinished mimetic business', in terms of unresolved conflicts along the fusion/separation axis, of absences and possessions, of battles to the death among contrasting Personae. It can also become a mirror that reflects the inadequacy of one's performances and the fallacy of one's interpretations.

The fact that this is experienced within (or alongside) a process that is nothing but a fiction, introduces the possibility of distance. Dramatic action is founded upon rules that are the same rules of life, but it puts them, so to say, 'in brackets', allowing us to observe it and to understand it without becoming too involved. In the meantime, however, it involves us, it transports us, it allows us to share emotions with another person (with the real other, the actor behind the mask), which, even though they are not real emotions (but *in a fiction*), they speak with the same voice. The dramatic play is a play of encounter.

Part II

Foundations of dramatherapy

Through the dramatic act, the actual embodiment of imaginative constructs through enacting them in front of an audience, an infinity of possibilities can be brought to life, and therefore witnessed and experienced.

(Grainger and Duggan 1997)

Elements

PLAY

On the shores of the ocean of the universe
Children have a feast.
   In the sky the storm is coming,
   In the sea the boat is sinking:
The angel of death passes flying,
Children keep on playing.
On the shores of the ocean of the universe
A great feast of children!
            (R. Tagore, *Sissu*, 1903)

Imagination and devotion

Not a long time ago, taking my 3-year-old little daughter V to her room to get her favourite puppet, I saw her suddenly become stiff – her arms leaning on the bed, with a strange smile on her face – and remain still for some time. When I asked her what she was doing she loosened from that position, telling me, 'I played I was dummy.'

The first thing she tells me with this sentence is that she is marking out a frame: *I was playing*. An eccentric attitude that may appear strange in an everyday context (and even worrying, as it could be considered a symptom) is being legitimized as play. In the world of play, a physical action takes on a different meaning. It refers to something else; it is an acted metaphor. The gesture of the child is a mimetic gesture – in the sense that it imitates the immobility of the doll – but it hints at other possibilities. The doll is an object that can come to life and take part in the stories of the world, but it can also be abandoned and even destroyed. Its coming to life, and being kept alive, can be produced only by an action of imagination sustained by a form of devotion, the gesture of turning toward and taking care.

Isn't it perhaps the same process allowing the birth of human children? Her mother and I had held her in our imagination long before she was born into the world. Imagining her – as a person of her own – allowed us to be able to contain her within us and to turn towards her. The same happened in our relationship. We each imagined the other immersed in this tide of change, and we took care of one another. The others can exist only if we are able to imagine and to love them.

Winnicott suggests that play is a route for the construction of the other inside us. The first movements of the child that will evolve in play are akin to those of other mammals: rolling, grabbing and following. So children begin a journey that will bring them to the motion's control, and therefore to conceive themselves as separate entities, that is the first sense of the body-self. Schilder's *body image*, far from being an achievement, in a cognitive mode, of the age in which language is developed, is something that starts emerging at the beginning of life, in a 'pre-reflexive and nonthematic' way, and keeps growing along with time, until it becomes the core of self-awareness. This process of becoming more and more individual, through an increasing separation from the background, sometimes comes to a crisis that might be painful. Some help may be needed to go through it. The transitional object, object of imagination and devotion, allows us to pass through one of these crises, which will end (if we find no obstacles) with the recognition of a relationship. Relationship is the ability to transcend the dichotomy of fusion/separation with a middle course, considering self separated from others, but also connected to them. The tragic truth of the Aristotelian principle that *A is not Not-A* is not denied, but another point of view is added, a point of view which includes a wide range of possibilities. I can recognize parts of myself in the other-than-me and this recognition is mutual. I can take care of the other and the other can take care of me. Each one can experience approaching and departing, without fear of losing themselves in either direction.

In V's calling for a witness to her pretence to be the dummy, she was celebrating the world of relationship.

Dramatic play

As we have seen, there is a strong affinity between play and drama, in the sense that both arise from the construction of a frame, establishing a separate and distinguishable space/time in comparison to the continuum of the things of the world. This space/time is a metaphoric one. It allows the opening of a range of possibilities of sense through actions that, on the one hand, evokes other actions in the world and, on the other hand, while making them essential, makes them universal, and discloses many other potential meanings. In the space of *as if*, the patterns through which, paraphrasing Goodman, we 'see and build worlds' are extraordinarily similar to those on which the making of interpersonal relationships proceeds.

Sue Jennings made up an outstanding descriptive model for play, working out Peter Slade's concepts that define mainly two kinds of play, according to the used medium: *Personal Play* and *Projected Play*. In Jennings's model, child's dramatic play goes through three phases of development, evolving one from another. Jennings calls this model 'the EPR Paradigm'. In the first phase, the *Embodiment* (somehow corresponding to Piaget's *sensomotory stage*), physicality is predominant in play. Children express their experience of the world, therefore primarily of the relationship with the mother, through the movement, the bodily tone and the senses. The body dramatizes the relationship: a child's body supports mother cradling it, but it can also engage and withstand her. In the *Projection* phase, children use the external objects in the construction of their symbolic world, attributing to them metaphoric meanings connected both with their affective and cognitive processes. The transitional object comes into contact with other symbolic objects, founding a relational universe:

> As the child moves beyond the immediate sensory experience of the toys, more complicated scenarios begin to emerge, cat feels poorly, clown is hungry, the doll's house is used to tell a story, teddy and rabbit go to the seaside.
>
> (Jennings 1998: 55)

The third phase, *Role*, is the one in which play becomes theatre: children can enact the other – whether it is real or fantastic – while still remaining themselves. They experience the dramatic paradox, transcending the Aristotelian principle of identity: to be *and* not to be at the same time:

> the paradoxical relationship between an actor and a role, a person and a Persona. When an actor, such as Vivien Leigh, takes on a role, such as Scarlett O'Hara, she is both herself (Leigh) and not herself (Scarlett) at the same time. In a like manner, a child playing

doctor is both the child (not-doctor) and the doctor (not-child) at the same time.

(Landy 1995: 8)

The 'let's pretend' creates a shared theatrical frame – with no audience – whose rules can be renegotiated in any moment. At the same time, children 'acquire a new way of seeing, both flexible and rigid, which can be translated later in life, when they realize that in a certain sense the behaviour can be bound to a logical type or to a style' (Bateson 1956: 35).

It could be interesting, at this point, to trace an analogy between the phases of dramatic play outlined in Jennings's model and some dramatic forms which might be defined as native. We easily find them mixed; nonetheless, considered as concepts, they can provide a possible general classification of the dramatic forms. The first phase, *Embodiment*, can be connected with those forms of performance that keep the actor's body as the symbolic centre of the expression. In the oriental theatre, and in general in almost all the extra-Western theatrical traditions, dramatic action is mainly encoded movement, often rhythmic and with a strong connection with the music, with a slight and often external use of words, nevertheless implying a narrative dimension (as in our classical ballet). The phase called *Projection* by Jennings, where objects are animated through their manipulation, is related to the area conventionally named *Figure Theatre*, in which puppets, marionettes and dolls of various types are employed, as well as silhouettes used in shadow theatre.

The third phase, *Role*, pivots on acting, on becoming someone else, and is relevant to modern Western theatre. While in the other theatrical forms action and story are in the foreground, character is at the very centre of it. In the whole modern Western theatre, dramaturgy spins around the complexity of the single character's soul. Somehow, we have behind us a tradition of more than three centuries – from Shakespeare to Čecov – of psychological theatre long before science started to deal with the soul's description. Setting the heart of drama in the vicissitudes of the individual soul, through the encounter with the others, it is relatively rare in the extra-European theatrical traditions.

We must consider the increasing importance given to the centrality of the individual in Western thought since the Renaissance, culminating in Romanticism (and in the birth of psychology as an autonomous discipline severed both from philosophy and from physiology). In his impressive study of comparative mythology, *The Masks of God*, Joseph Campbell (1959/1969) tells us how, since the late Middle Ages, when the epics of chivalry turned into the adventure of the soul in the world, mythological thought has come increasingly to turn toward humanness rather than the supernatural, focusing on the psychological rather than on the religious sphere. This mythology of the individual, named by Campbell *creative mythology*, exalts the transformative strength of the human being, rooting in the deep zones of the soul, which reconnect us with what Giordano Bruno called *Anima Mundi*, the soul of the world.

The mythological/spiritual sphere of the individual, seen by Campbell mainly as expressed in art,[1] has been put under siege by two opposite and complementary tendencies peculiar to the technological-industrial societies: isolation and standardization. Isolation is the rarefaction of meaningful, affectively connoted relationships, more and more confined into small family nuclei, often with a mistrustful attitude towards the others. The corporate level is delegated to the institutions (for instance, in the area of childhood and adolescence to the school); the feeling of *communitas*, of the sharing among human beings of values and common objectives, is fragmented in a system of affiliations to circles, lobbies and subcultures, often potentially xenophobic. Standardization produces an identification of the individual's value system with pre-existent existential models. The personal mythologies of success, appearance and possessions often lead the life of the individuals to an unsatisfied tension toward an unattainable goal, generating a sense of failure and frustration that produces, in a perverse recursive circuit, further isolation and sometimes illness and extreme behaviours. Even the child's play is threatened by these tendencies, with the break-in of the structured technological toy, to be used in solitude, demanding a rigid use that limits the possible spaces of imagination. On the other hand, the imaginative structures produced as commodities by mass media, often with the advice of experts shamelessly exploiting their psychological knowledge with intents of manipulation and business, penetrate our children's imagination, conditioning the freedom of their play.

Fortunately, play withstands. There are certainly many adults who work hard to protect it, but I believe that children's resources for creating their world and themselves, for building the other and the relationship – resources that are expressed through play – are inexhaustible. I have seen nursery school children playing Pokémons[2] and devising an amazing range of variations, which gave everyone the space to invent – and to invent themselves in relationship with the others.

The recovery of this quality of dramatic play as experimentation in the world of the relationship, fostering the growth and expansion of individual identity, is a foundational hypothesis of Dramatherapy.

Order and chaos

The experimentation with identity and relationship in play is creative in the sense that it doesn't establish hypotheses to be verified (or eventually to be falsified), as happens in scientific thought (or at least in its formalization, which has served as a model for many theories of learning), but it stirs on impulse, building and redefining itself during its very movement. It is, in a sense, a process of the kind defined by Bateson (1979), stochastic, combining randomness with a selection that leads to the permanence of some elements. A primary selective criterion is the player's satisfaction, the pleasure and joy of the realization. These feelings can be evoked by the variety and wealth of the experimented possibilities, or by the harmony of the forms that play allows to rise, or by the dynamics of tension/release within the process. They are very similar to the aesthetical feelings, to the 'great shiver', that shakes people creating a work of art and people enjoying it.

In his *Homo Ludens*, which is probably the most acute reflection on play made during last century, Johan Huizinga has written:

> The play in itself, although it is an activity of the spirit, doesn't contain a moral function, either virtue, or sin. If therefore the play is not connected directly with the truth, nor with the good, can it be perhaps found in the dominion of the beauty, then? Here our judgment hesitates. Beauty is not inherent to the play as such, yet it has a tendency to bind itself to various elements of it. Gentleness and grace are connected since the beginning with the most primitive forms of play. [. . .] In its more evolved forms, play is interwoven with rhythm and harmony, the noblest quality of the aesthetic perceptive faculty that is given to man. The ties between play and beauty are manifold and firm.
>
> (Huizinga 1939: 10–11)

Play, art, beauty: in these words is contained the idea of a tension between order and chaos, between form and vagueness, between continuous and discrete, between balance and imbalance. According to Huizinga:

> Within the spaces destined to play, a proper and absolute order is dominating. And here's a new and more positive sign of play: it creates an order, it is order. It realizes in the defective world and in the confused life a temporary, limited perfection.
>
> (ibid.: 14)

With play, a new order appears through the break-up and the shaking of the previous one, an order that can be recognized as such even if it is different from the other one, and that reveals itself crossing the chaos; it is an enrichment of sense that transforms and allows understanding. This tension between order/chaos is characteristic of the ritual process. Victor Turner, in his seminal study on ritual/theatre connections, starting from the descriptive model of the rites of passage elaborated by Arnold Van Gennep (1909), calls *liminal phenomena* those which I have called threshold phenomena in the previous chapter, and dwells upon the social value of the rite as a collective event that refounds the community. But this refoundation happens through a passage in the chaos:

> Liminality is a temporal interface, whose properties are the partial overturn of those of the already consolidated arrangement on which is founded any specific cultural 'cosmos'.
>
> (Turner 1982: 94)

There are modes of ritual nearer to the polarity of chaos, leaning toward agitation and movement, lack of moderation and excess, drunkenness and trance. Others privilege instead form and completeness, rule and control. In every case the ritual process includes in itself the presence and integration of opposite polarities, both Dionysian and Apollonian. Roger Caillois, reflecting on the presence of this polarity in play, calls one of the poles *paidia*, marked by:

> a common principle of fun, turbulence, free improvisation and a light-hearted vital fullness. At the opposite extremity, this restless and spontaneous exuberance is almost totally absorbed, and however disciplined, by a complementary tendency, opposite, under certain aspects but not at all, to its anarchic and capricious nature: an increasing demand to subdue it to some arbitrary, mandatory, intentionally hindering conventions.
>
> (Caillois 1967: 29)

Caillois calls this aspect of play *ludus*. In theatre, the direction is generally from chaos to order, from experimentation to form, from anarchy to rule. In play, and in dramatic play particularly, the relationship of order/chaos spins around a rather dynamic pattern,[3] an alternation of the opposite trends, mutually generating each other, and mutually holding the one up on the other, continually producing novelty that can be shared in virtue of their conversion in forms.

The dramatic group processes in Dramatherapy develop along this dynamic pattern. They provide moments in which chaos and confusion are absolute, allowing us to learn to face the uncertainties and moments of loss of control over things that so frequently occur in our lives; but at the same time they are moments of origin, of *status nascendi*, of creative imbalance from which, through a process of arrangement that leads to form and communication, new structures can emerge.

To learn again to play can be a difficult task, involving the embarrassment of feeling childish or the sense of shame coming from devoting our time to activities that society stigmatizes as useless. However, if it is sustained by a climate of trust and liking, it produces a possible way in to the refreshing experience of a shared creative play. In play, as Grainger writes:

> people's fear of being caught off guard and not knowing what to do, their painful inability to 'join in', are overcome by satisfaction of having something to do that doesn't really matter ('after all, it's only a game') and that no-one does very well. If it makes people laugh, so much the better.
>
> (Grainger 1995: 36)

NARRATIVE

> God created man because He likes stories.
> (Elie Wiesel, *The Doors of the
> Forest*, 1964)

Stories of stories

This is a story I have already told elsewhere,[4] but I am pleased to tell it again now and I think it could be useful.

Once, on a winter evening many years ago, I found my two children, 3-year-old A and 5-year-old M, hidden under the blankets. I could hear little shouts and laughter, the bed squeaking under the movements of a small well-hidden mass of children under two layers of soft wool. When I saw a little head peeping out, I asked: 'What are you doing?' And they answered: 'We are playing Pinocchio.'

Their night adventure was a descent into obscurity, a challenge to the great fear, the fear of the darkness, that is the fear of the unknown, of the mysterious sea under which monsters are concealed, of the evening shade in which the traveller hastens. A protected challenge, in this case, in a place where we feel safe, and in company. The bed, which was once a place where the first separation was celebrated, and has then become a safe territory of shelter and protection, for a while turns into the stage of a nightly journey toward the heart of our restlessness.

> My bed is like a little boat;
>   Nurse helps me in when I embark;
> She girds me in my sailor's coat
>   And starts me in the dark.
>
> [. . .]
>
> All night across the dark we steer;
>   But when the day returns at last,
> Safe in my room, beside the pier,
>   I find my vessel fast.
> (Robert Louis Stevenson, *My Bed is a Boat*, 1906)

The comic strip 'Little Nemo in Slumberland' by Winsor McCay (a masterpiece of twentieth-century visionary art, I maintain) tells of the nightly trips of a child invited by the Princess of the Dreams' Country to visit the kingdom. Often Nemo's departures happen through a metamorphosis of the bed that soars, sinks, or is provided with legs and starts running, or lengthens up to the sky.

In the case of my children, this ambivalence between safety and fear, between the thrill of the not known and the safety of the already known, becomes a shared game because it tells a story. If I say 'Let's slip under the blankets and pretend to be afraid', I am shaping a structure. If I say 'Let's play Pinocchio', I am inviting you to enter an image. The narrative dimension allows the meeting of the imaginations around a nucleus of strong symbolic tension. The story of Pinocchio's amazing journey inside the belly of the whale in search of his lost father, resounding mythical themes, is gently borrowed to give a clear sense to the play, allowing also to present it to a non-player. At the same time the story recreates the play, enriching it with symbolic echoes that can be intuitively caught and putting it in another time and space, which can be explored imaginatively.

I cannot exclude that in my telling this story once again, other stories are concealed: the story, for instance, of my growth and of my personal search for the father, or the search for my being, in my turn, a father to creatures that are both mine and not mine.[5] But that is another story.

Thinking by stories

Gregory Bateson, in *Mind and Nature*, tells us the following story (warning the reader that he has already reported it elsewhere):

> A man wanted to know the mind, not in nature, but, on the contrary, in a big personal computer. He asked it (perhaps in his more polished Fortran): 'Do you estimate that you will ever think as a human being?' Then the machine got down to work, analysing its own habits of calculation; it finally printed the answer on a sheet of paper, as these machines usually do. The man ran to see the answer and found, clearly printed, the following words: THIS REMINDS ME OF A STORY.
>
> (Bateson 1979: 27–8)

To tell stories and to listen to them is a prominent activity in human communication. I can tell a story to exemplify a concept; to express an opinion or to solicit one from my listener; to consolidate a bond of belonging between teller and listener; to bring to the other's knowledge information about me or about the world. These motivations often coexist and are intertwined. Sometimes I have come across a group of people that remembered a departed friend. Stories are added to stories, and everyone tells a personal experience lived with the remembered friend, and everyone comes to discover facts of his life and aspects of his personality that were ignored. This weaving of stories and feelings creates a warm feeling of community that helps us to bear the basic truth that all these stories reveal: the impermanence and frailty of human things. Or, to tell another story, I currently work in a care and rehabilitation centre for teenagers with personality disorders. The staff gather once a week to talk about clients, to appraise the progress of the therapeutic process and to calibrate our work toward a greater effectiveness. A good part of the meeting time (which can last more than four hours) is devoted to telling stories about the boys and girls, and of ourselves in relation to them. We recall the events that have happened during the days, within the creative workshops or in more informal moments; their stories of home and school; the stories of their families; the stories, real or imagined, that they tell of themselves or about themselves, and even the stories of fiction (movies and cartoons) they like the best. Every so often, time is not enough for telling everything, and the stories continue to mill around, at the end of the work day or during the breaks. They form a common awareness, encouraging us to sharpen our sensibility for helping our clients to help themselves. The stories we exchange verify or disprove our hypotheses. They enhance the knowledge we have of our clients and the images we have of them. Finally, they support us as a common culture, more intuitively powerful than a thousand theories, in the difficult task of the helping relationship. Moreover, it might have happened to anyone, in a country house during a rainy evening, or around the fire of a summer camp, to experience the pleasure of a shiver of fear while telling and hearing ghost stories. Here the fanciful tale exorcizes the anxious presence of natural forces so much greater than us, and it connects us one to another in the shared imagination. Like the narrators of Boccaccio's *Decameron*, telling stories in which countless aspects of human nature – wisdom and foolishness, hate and love, holiness and perversion, violence and tenderness – weave a cheerful dance, they claim the power of life upon death impending everywhere.

Someone could object that the stories in the examples I have just given are not the same kind of stories. Some are real-life stories; others are products of the imagination (fictional). The sociologist Paolo Jedlowski (2000) calls these narrative modes 'the pole of Testimony and the pole of Fabulation', but he warns:

> To say 'poles' means that they are the extreme positions of the expression of two tensions that animate the field of the narration. In concrete, the stories that we tell are usually placed within a continuum between these poles, participating in different measure of both the tensions.
>
> (Jedlowski 2000: 40)

In every story told, both these polarities are present.[6] If I tell a story that really happened to me, I will exalt some details and skip others; I will lengthen or shorten the time; I will paint with emotional hues of some aspects. In brief, even if my aim is pure objectivity, with no purpose of deception, my story will be interwoven with fiction, and so much more if it is far away in time. On the other hand, if I devise a story, even with the simple purpose of entertaining someone, this story is mine nonetheless, and parts of myself, of my imaginary world and of my experience of things, are held and expressed. In every story told, whether it stands on the side of Testimony or on the side of Fabulation, I tell both about myself and about the world.

Narrative identity

In his remarkable film *Mahābhārata*, Peter Brook enshrines the immense Indian epic poem inside a narrative frame. In the first scene of the film drawn from the play, a boy wanders in the labyrinths of a temple cavern, by the light of countless candles. Amazed, he crosses richly ornamented halls, with many masks on the walls and trays full of offerings, and finally he enters the darkest aisles, where he comes across an old man, sitting in deep meditation. At the presence of the boy, the man opens his eyes. He looks at him and asks him if he knows how to write. 'No', answers the boy, astounded. 'Why?'

Getting up and coming close to him, the man explains, 'I have composed a great poem. It is complete, but there is nothing written of it. I need someone to write what I know.'

'What's your name?'

'Vyasa.'

'What's your poem about?'

'You.'

'Me?'

'Yes, it is the story of your kind, of the birth of your ancestors, how they grew up, and of the terrible war that derived from it. It is the poetic history of mankind. If you listen to it carefully, at the end you will be another person.' At this point Ganeša, the elephant-headed god, master of the categories, appears, and offers himself as a scribe. So the story can start.

In the poem, the story is told by a narrator; even better there are two narrators, one of whom tells about the telling other. The intuition of Brook to identify the teller of the story that will be performed with Vyasa, the legendary author of the poem (the Indian Homer), therefore combining narrator and author of the story in a single character, emphasizes the creative aspect of the teller, who gives life to the world while telling it. But this creation can be done only by virtue of two factors: first, that it is comprehensible. The guarantor of this is Ganeša who, as master of the categories, represents 'the principle of every classification that allows us to establish a relationship among different orders of things between the macrocosm and the microcosm' (Daniélou 1992). He authorizes the knowledge (which, according to Bateson, we can only define as knowledge of differences and relationships).

The second factor is perhaps more important: someone listening is necessary so that the story comes to life – another human being. The relationship with another human being is different from the relationship with things. Martin Heidegger maintained that people *take care* of things, but *have care* of other people. Therefore a basic be-with (*mitdasein*) is inherent to the nature of human beings. It may be hidden under heaps of distrust, disaffection and fear, but it is there anyway, and at times we find some ways to unearth it again and allow it to unfold in a generous consonance with the other beings. One of these ways is by telling stories. While telling and listening to stories, we are building together, narrator and listener, a form of co-existence:

> The great quality of the narrator, the lesson that can be drawn by his work is this: a narrator is in direct contact with his public. Conditions are very simple: there is a person who knows a story and there are some people looking and longing to enter the secret, hidden world of his imagination.
>
> (Peter Brook, quoted in Di Bernardi 1989: 141)

First of all, people telling open a door that allows a meeting with something that belongs to their inner world, and that concerns them. Until I have told it, a story is mine and only mine. The very moment I tell it, it becomes everybody's story.[7] Nonetheless, stories play an important part in the making of people as individuals.

Jean-Claude Carrière, who worked with Brook at the *Mahābhārata*'s dramaturgy, collected together a lot of traditional stories he found during the many journeys with the company. In his introduction to the book, he underscores, in a charming poetic language, the connection between narrative and personal identity:

> We are nothing but stories. And without story, without possibility to tell this story, we are not at all or we are little. And as a story is mostly movement from a point to the other, movement that never leaves the things in the initial state, so we live in this continuous flow, in this mutability. There is for us a beginning, there will be an end.
>
> (Carrière 1998: 10)

Achieving this awareness is perhaps the only viable choice between a desperate grasping to a 'strong core' of the 'I', increasingly put under siege by cultural sea-changes, and letting oneself go to the play of *multiphrenia*, emptying the concept of personal identity of its function as a primary element of our being in the world. The notion of *narrative identity*, first enunciated by Paul Ricoeur, does not deny versatility and mutability, but redefines it within an interaction between *sameness* and *ipseity*. *Sameness* refers to identity as *idem*: the unaltered permanence of a substance in time; *ipseity* to identity as *ipse*: keeping a continuity throughout a flow of change by the sense of keeping a promise. The result of this interaction can be described in narrative terms: the dialectics of *character* and *plot* can bestow significance to the concept of identity. They mutually found each other:

> We understand the *character*'s identity transferring upon him the operation of construction of the *plot*, first applied to the action told; the *character* itself is construed within the *plot*.
>
> (Ricoeur 1990: 234)

Goethe wrote to his friend Schiller, who had questioned the poet about the meaning of his *Das Märchen* (which means simply 'fairytale'), the following words: 'There are more than twenty characters in the story. What are they all doing? Nothing but the story, my dear.' The construction of identity passes through stories and our mirroring in them:

> Persons designate themselves as narrative unity of a life – life reflecting the dialectics of cohesion and dispersion exhibited by the plot.
>
> (Ricoeur 1992: 68)

Our stories relate with others' stories, and this relationships generates new meanings, but the encounter with the other is also engendered by fiction: 'Fiction is a vast field of experiment for the endless job of identification we do for ourselves' (Ricoeur 1992: 69).

Playing with time

The play dimension, as we have seen, sets up a special frame, cutting it out of the everyday space/time; a frame in which all the events are endowed with a special significance. So indeed the narrative dimension brings the possibility of a refoundation of time, not only in the sense that the story develops structuring itself as a sequence of linked events, but also and above all because, in virtue of the powerful presence of a component of fiction, it allows the actual quality of time as a project to be revealed. Time narrated is time built, not only measured (as St Augustine remarks) by the soul. In the telling of stories, time is unfolded not as absolute and irreversible, but as a pattern of possibility, and we are in a condition to dwell in each of them. A story told in the space of play: this is drama. Quoting Brook again:

I think that there is no contradiction between illusion and not-illusion. A good narrator creates an imaginary world, the listener believes him and, if the narrator is really good, he believes him in the one hundred percent; but at the same time he never loses sight of the fact that he is a narrator. In a satisfactory and totally tension-free way, there is a double vision: the teller is seen and imagination is seen as well. For me this is always what makes theatre beautiful and effective.

(in Di Bernardi 1989: 148)

A story told in Dramatherapy can develop in innumerable actions, each one endowed with a slightly different meaning. It can be also repeated, but can never be identical; it can be coloured with countless different colours. In the moment when the narration becomes performance, the *fabula* becomes action, the story opens to an active mirroring. Entering with my body inside the narration, I participate in it, making it, in its mimetic resonances, a community event. Relationship among people through imagination is enriched by presence, and the energy of the multiplicity is embodied in my interpretation/performance. In this sense, the narrative dimension reaffirms the principle of the freedom and power that we exert over our destiny as human beings able to think and to imagine.

ROLE

Ah! The paths are all in me.
Whatever distance, direction, or term
Belongs to me, it's me. The rest is the part
Of me that I call the external world.
But the path – my god – here is now bifurcating
In who I am and in the other from me.
(F. Pessoa, *Poems*, 1942)[8]

Roles to play

At the age of two my little daughter V decided to begin to speak, and she has not stopped since then. Besides setting questions, asking for help, expressing surprise and wonder, she comments with words upon all of her own actions. On a summer afternoon, with a soft lukewarm wind blowing, slightly scented, I unrolled a straw mat on the lawn, aiming to lie down and relax. As soon as V saw the scene, she approached walking on all fours and huddled just in the middle of the mat, with an attitude of great enjoyment. Then she lifted her head toward me, looking at me with a cheeky expression, and said, 'I am a small dog.' I simply crouched close to her saying, 'And I am a big dog.' The child seized the opportunity, and turned to me with a small bark. And so the play began. Since then, at least a part of the time I spend with her has been devoted to the 'small dog and big dog' game. At the beginning, the small dog mainly asked for cuddles, then for nourishment and care. Then, the two dogs started to play, just like dogs do, with a ball or a twig, and afterwards they began explorations and adventures, like hunting wolves in the forest. At times we changed animal, maintaining, however, the proportions (small wolf and big wolf, small elephant and big elephant). At times the roles were reversed for a little while; I acted as the small dog and she was the big one. But most of the time, small dog and big dog simply built some ways of being among the things of the world, commenting on them from a position of liberty: together with 'big dog' so many things can be done, not only because he protects me, but also, and above all, because as I can invent being a dog, I can invent the world too.

Our father–daughter relationship was enlightened by a metaphor. Though remaining as a background to the play, a point of reference that firmly connects us with reality, and therefore also a strong affective container, in the world of the metaphor it shows itself as a broadening of the whole range of possibilities. This enrichment can subsist in virtue of some characteristics of the context connected to general themes we have analysed before.

First, we are moving inside imagination. Many layers of knowledge are necessary to come to a statement such as 'I am a small dog', layers that contain differences and analogies. I must have learned to distinguish between me and the surrounding world, and therefore between me and the other. I must also know that I am more similar to some beings than to others and I must somehow build up the awareness that I belong to a species (human rather than canine). This operation must not have been easy, considering that V has learned to crawl surrounded by various animals (dogs and cats) stirring around her at her own height. There is, then, a similarity between me and them, as they are as small as me, more or less, and walk the same way I walk, and there is a similarity between me and these people taking care of me. Then, having gained the erect position, I can begin to understand that there are deeper similarities to an extent unlike the morphological one, involving the level of the behavioural structures, for example, in the play intercourse between an adult animal and a pup. Somehow I am *like* a dog. But if I say 'I am a dog' the analogy is turned into metaphor, and this can happen only in virtue of an imaginative leap, which, as we have seen before, not only makes present the absent, but endows it with sense and life on its own. Imagination connects in a single figure the whole range of differences and analogies, making this figure dynamic and liable to experiments and transformations. These experiments and transformations that – and this is the second aspect – can be acted only within the respect of a relational mutuality. The imaginative roles we interpret/perform, co-exist mutually sustaining each other. The one without the other has little sense, or has a completely different one: it's quite a different matter if I imagine being a small dog in relationship with a place, a desert, for instance. Co-existence means a dynamic equilibrium built together. It means to influence the other and be influenced by them in turn (Martin Buber's *sphere of the interhuman*). In musical terms it could be compared to J. S. Bach's counterpoint, in which the musical themes converse and weave, mutually modifying each other, at times developing side by side, at times building together something new.

The third aspect is the fact that the role (even within a relationship being to some extent the pre-existing form of it) is a free choice. The father and daughter roles are pre-set, both by a biological fact and by a cultural one. They are, of course, modulated upon an infinity of individual variables, but the basic condition remains: the sharing of a type of relationship that founds the human community. Variations and elaborations are feasible, but limited in number and extension. The imaginative role is taken on, instead, with a deliberate action, and it encloses the dimension of freedom. Inside the frame of play everything is possible: to test out both the other and oneself, for instance; to experiment with the limits of affect and fear; to cross the land of uncertainty and to get out of it as a winner.

Imagination, coexistence, choice: as the universality of the relationship is embodied in the particular and disclosed in it, it becomes plentiful with potential meanings. Taking and playing roles, the human being 'stands open to a revealing restructuring of his humanity, a restructuring to which he allows free experimental play for the moment' (Wilshire 1982: 105).

Person, Persona, role

At this point it is necessary to take a step backwards to clarify the concept of Role, which I have already used without going thoroughly into it. We have used the Jungian notion of Persona to define the particular form that individuals assume in their social presentation, which has the characteristic of being an interface between the internal and external world, and the tendency to conform itself to already fixed cultural models. We have underlined the tendency of the Persona to impose itself as a dominant structure, suppressing other important aspects of the individual soul, and therefore limiting the expression of its potentialities in the world; and also as a protective tool against the emotional threats coming from the others' world.

Going back to the etymology, we can notice that, even if both terms are derived from theatre, there is a difference between them. Persona reminds us of the mask, with suggestive associations concerning its use in the rite as a sign of the presence of the other (the God), which is a total presence, signified in the event by the loss of identity of the one wearing it (Plato's *divine folly*).

Role draws its origin from the Latin *rotulus*, which is the name of the roll of paper or vellum upon which the actor's part was written. Role makes us think, therefore, of a prescribed sequence of behaviour – words, gestures, expressions, bodily attitudes and other communication signs – coherent with a definition of the character moving within given circumstances. In this sense we can say that Role is a more restrictive and, at the same time, more comprehensive concept than that of Persona. Restrictive since, while Persona refers to a construction investing the whole expression of the individual in the world, shaping itself as a unity endowed with some coherence, Role describes a segment of this expression, a complex typical behaviour related to a specific situation and to particular relationships active in that situation. Comprehensive since, as roles are related to specific relational contexts, therefore to a condition of change rather than of stability, they can include a wide range of expressions and are liable to change.

George Herbert Mead's (1934) book, *Mind, Self and Society*, was one of the first, though uncertain, attempts to build a dramatic theory of the personality. According to him, taking on a role (experimenting therefore through being in another's shoes, with the other's point of view) is not only the root of the possibility of intersubjective relationships, but also of the building of the self. In Mead's conception, role can be defined as connected with relationship, or even seen as a function of a relationship. Every role can exist only in a relationship of mutual dependence with a counter-role that can be embodied by an individual or by a group. Yet the counter-role can be also imaginary, as in the case of paranoia, of which we talked before. However, even what Mead calls taking on a role, the experience of feeling what the other feels (or at least what we imagine the other feels)[9] has an imaginative as well as mimetic component. As an imaginative action, it demands that the sharing be confirmed, and not distorted or destroyed.

The role is therefore a manifestation of the Persona in the relational here and now, but since it can exist only in a dynamic process of relationship, it contradicts the rigidity of the Persona, introducing into it the dimension of versatility. This can obviously happen only in those cases when access to the writing of the script is guaranteed to the individual.

Role as a creative pattern

Role has therefore both a prescriptive aspect, connected to the mimetic construction of the Persona, and a flexible one, connected to the relational event: once more a rigid model and a pattern of possibility are facing each other. To confine oneself to a rigid model can be a necessity, when the individual lacks the essential resources to govern flexibility. Flexibility means actually to relinquish some safety, first of all the centring of the self. To leave a walled construction of identity for an imbalance that allows going toward the other means to be exposed to innumerable threats. Opening the emotional channels, for instance, reveals our own frailty, and leads to the risk of entering an uncontrollable emotional stream. We run the risk of being under the others' sway, in the sense of allowing the others to enter my world unconditionally, imposing their rules. A rigid role, not admitting any loosening (that is, exasperatingly coherent), immediately identifiable and thinkable, can be a good watchdog.

For some years I have been leading drama workshops within a social project aimed at preventing youth delinquency in a marginal district of Palermo: the ZEN district, acronym freely interpreted by the local teenagers as *Zona Elementi Nocivi* (harmful elements zone), while it actually means a less picturesque *Zona Espansione Nord* (north expansion zone). I remember that my first 'warm' welcome to the district was the cutting of all four tyres of my car. I had been recommended to adopt a, so to say, 'ethological' strategy in my approach to this reality: show them immediately who is the boss, otherwise they will trample on you. Anyway, if you can tell from the start what it is going to be like, I could not expect an easy life. I have to admit that 'playing the tough one' was the guarantee for a survival space and made the boys respect me (though respect is, in the Sicilian culture, essentially the recognition of a hierarchy, a 'pecking order'). Something didn't work. I succeeded in maintaining a certain order and in guaranteeing that there were no transgressions in the group (at least in my presence), but it was as if that attitude, ranging from collaboration to subjection, and suppressing the expressions of open rebellion, was somewhat artificial. There was something behind it (a suffering, perhaps?) that could not be revealed. The role of the subordinate, recognizing the power of someone stronger than him, but longing to rebel at the bottom of his heart, was sadly for them a very well-known role, inscribed in a culture imbued with what Leonardo Sciascia called *mafia feeling*. However, was I able to afford to give up such protection and to go around without an escort? We were, they and me, trapped in roles that were complementary and symmetrical at the same time: nothing could happen in that stiffened equilibrium – nothing bad, of course, but also nothing good. The role of the tough one began to bore me, conflicting as it was with my personal inclination towards an educational approach founded on gentleness. I decided that I might be able to play it with some detachment, a sort of Brechtian *estrangement*, which *showed* instead of *being*, not wearing out my emotional supplies but serving the purpose as well. I realized that this condition, this acting style, allowed me to separate the authority necessary for keeping order from a more empathic position, in which I could set myself to listening to their hidden feelings. They perceived this shifting of style, interpreting it not as a yielding of borders but as a chance to approach. The roles at first so rigidly symmetrical, started to become permeable, influencing each other through a mutual transformation, to a point in which protective rigidity became unnecessary and emotions began to flow freely.

This process of loosening and restructuring produced two amazing effects: the boys and girls started to speak about themselves (and their misdeeds) and also started to act. While acting, they could experience many role variations, in a review of existential pluralities that did not exclude being 'harmful elements', but can envisage a whole lot of different possibilities. As for me, I can say that this metamorphosis contributed to release a tension, allowing me to become more and more open to meet experiences of the world different from mine, dipping into them in order to understand them 'from inside', though keeping a distance that allowed me to observe, analyse and appraise.

Moreno's thinking focused on this double significance of role. He speaks of *canned roles* to define those fixed, culturally conditioned strategies of behaviour that everyone sets up in interpersonal situations, more or less like Goffman's *presentations of self*. These roles sometimes have a certain amount of social effectiveness, but what they miss is the creative dimension, which, according to Moreno, is intimately connected with a specific quality of the person that he calls *spontaneity*. Moreno's concept of spontaneity is somewhat vague, defined in poetic, rather than scientific, language:

The state of spontaneity is not permanent, it is not fixed and rigid as the written words or the melodies, but it is flowing, with a rhythmic fluency, that rises and falls, grows and fades like life's actions, yet it is different from life. It is the productive state, the essential principle of every creative experience.

(Moreno 1946: 134)

We can figure out Moreno's spontaneity as a concept akin to Jung's *libido* (psychic energy in a primary state) on the one hand, and to Henri Bergson's *élan vital* (organizing principle that embodies in the organic) on the other, or, with a hazardous but fascinating jump, to the Polynesian *mana* studied by Marcel Mauss (supernatural power showing itself in the human energy).

Jonathan Fox, the founder of Playback Theatre (which is Psychodrama's most theatrical offshoot), has attempted a more analytical description of spontaneity, considering the signs through which it is manifested. Fox (1986) states four of them, each having an internal, self-aware aspect validated by an external relational aspect. The first sign is *Vitality*, experienced by the subject as a feeling of fullness and vigour, a feeling of being 'in the flow'. This corresponds to being perceived as active, vital and able to transmit energy. The second sign is *Appropriateness*. Fox writes:

The idea of spontaneity as a heedless impulse belittles the potential of the concept, which can include a difficult-to-attain notion of 'right action', not unlike the Zen master's injunction to 'eat while eating, sleep while sleeping'.

(Fox 1986: 80)

Appropriateness is the feeling that our own actions and reactions are not false notes, but belong to a harmony of the relationship; they are fitting to the context and, meanwhile, they contribute to its construction and definition. A further sign is *Intuition*, the ability to interact with no thought mediation. This means a particular listening attitude toward the non-verbal and non-intentional signals of the communication, as well as a 'gestaltic' stance, allowing us to synthctically accept the moment, understanding it even before acknowledging it. The last element listed by Fox in his analysis is *Readiness for change*. Facing the unexpected means developing 'an ability to accept each moment as it comes, and respond dynamically' (ibid.). This facing mostly happens in the meeting with the other.

True spontaneity implies giving over the safety coming from a stubborn clinging to a rigid but solid configuration. Safety has to be sought in a position of acceptance of the mutability of things, in assuming change as a natural life quality.

Role constructs

In the intercourse with the other, a rigid role can impose the rules of the game, or it can conform to them. The spontaneous role can modify the rules of the game, or suggest new ones. In terms of Kelly's theory, a relationship entails the loosening of the tight role constructs, and their recomposition on the basis of the novelty introduced by the other.

A personal construct system, according to Kelly, is an organization of relationships between individual and world, structured through similarities and oppositions, sometimes nonthematic and therefore beyond the reach of consciousness. A construct is a 'world vision', a whole group of ideas, values and principles, consciously and hierarchically organized, but also a series of relational automatisms, with widespread emotional connotations, which are not thought and often not thinkable. Constructs arise as tools to move in the world, to foresee the events and therefore to act toward their improvement. When a construct works, it produces the tendency to be kept unchanged even when the contexts change, and it becomes ineffective. In this case it is necessary to loosen the constructs, to give room, so that similarities and differences, analogies and oppositions can be modified, including other possibilities not yet conceived. This passage can involve us in chaos and conflict, before new constructs emerge more attuned with the changed situations.

In the case of my ZEN story (intended again as district), my playing a strong powerful role as a prevention of impending aggressions was connected with a fear/challenge opposition that I had absorbed during my childhood while living in a district in which the ways of socialization were not so different from the ZEN ones, and which I believed I had left behind me in virtue of ideal and cultural choices. It was also connected with the distance/invasion opposition, which is, if well used, an excellent tool of the trade for the practitioner in the field of the 'helping relationship', but which, along with the other, composes a rigid defensive building. The possibility that the other side of distance can be empathy, for instance, would make more fluid the continuum between the two extremes and would allow a dynamic setting in it, but this possibility is blocked by the connection with the other opposition. If fear appears, there are very few alternatives: escape (which in my case would have meant giving up my job); subjection (which would clash with the educational task to which I had been assigned), or attack. Distance/attack marks a position of alarm and tension that is rather uncomfortable to hold for a long time. The remarkable thing is that this structure of oppositions was the same one that supported the behaviour of the young people I was with. But, though rigid, a role, in its general meaning, depends on the interpretations/ performances given by the unique actor. My conforming to that model, although not entirely conscious, was tempered by other elements: my beliefs and values, for instance, or my affective experience as a parent. These elements have influenced a change in interpretative style, opening the doors for humour, and humour is the best antidote for fear.

Parameters of the game

Role constructs, until they remain within the range of potentiality, until the roles are not played in the here and now of the relationship, are mostly *endocepts*. This term is used by Arieti to define:

> a primitive organization of experiences, perceptions, mnemonic traces, images of things and movements of the past. These previous experiences, removed and not brought to the consciousness, keep having an indirect influence. [. . .] The content of an *endocept* can be communicated to the others only when it is translated into expressions belonging to other levels: for example in words, music, sketches and so on.
>
> (Arieti 1976: 60–61)

Roles remain at the level of the *endocept* until they come into contact with some counter-roles that define them. This operation can be purely imaginative. I can mentally represent myself in a situation, and therefore I can build a hypothetical role. Yet roles, to be wholly accomplished, must come into play. When a role is played – that is, interpreted/performed – and linked to a context authorizing it (or else invalidating it), it takes a *form*, that is a sequence of behaviours visible to others as also to ourselves, and a *structure* (a system of meanings) that puts in relation the constructive and interpretative modes acted, and the answers to such modes. Grainger lists some remarkable parameters of this structure with reference to the interpretative modes and therefore to the tension of actor/role.

Awareness vs. unawareness

In everyday life we are not actively aware of the roles we play, apart from the roles played in situations in which the dramatic aspect is outstandingly marked (as in ceremonies, in law or politics, in working organizations). For the rest, we simply act in a way we perceive suitable to the situation:

> The social drama is experienced as a seamless matrix of action and interaction where figure and ground are in constant flux; where actors and audience are one.
>
> (Grainger and Duggan 1997: 54)

Every now and then we have to face new roles; in work, for instance, with a new charge of responsibility; or in the affective life when the sense of a relationship is modified by a status change, ratified by the community, with marriage or the birth of a child. Then, the awareness of a passage from one role to another emerges as necessity to construct the newness through the disarrangement of an identity balance already reached (seemingly, at least), and the making of a new one around the new necessities. But awareness itself can also be an obstacle in this process of restructuring. We become aware not only of some positive aspects related to the new role, but also of the difficulties, of the responsibilities, of the ties, as well as of the fact of having an audience observing us and waiting for our best possible performance. The excessive awareness becomes embarrassment, self-consciousness and worry; so often it leads us to inadequate performances. In contrast, a total lack of awareness prevents us from properly facing the new rules and the new potentialities, and therefore to modify our role in an evolving sense. To reconcile awareness with spontaneity is an artist's alchemy; the maximum of the awareness along with the maximum of spontaneity: the paradox of the art of the actor.

Complexity vs. simplicity

A role can be played on the basis of minimal elements, enough to connote it. The training of the American marines is centred upon clear rules, values and objectives, which are inculcated in recruits' minds by keeping them in a constant state of stress, and which conform the individual personality to a unique, essential role: that of the anonymous war machine. In Hollywood cinema, the characters of marines are often portrayed with a role parallel to what can be supposed to be the result of the training; a role that both reflects it and hides it: John Wayne's *Green Berets*, unbalanced on the side of values, are presented as heroes of the free world, men of sterling character, brave and aware of their mission. More problematic is the image shown in Stanley Kubrick's *Full Metal Jacket* of those bewildered young people, and the fierce role they are forced to learn, which cohabits with a mix of conflicting, deeply human feelings – fear and pride, boldness and weakness, nostalgia and sense of dismay, even madness – so that they become closer to us and more intimately true. There are, of course, moments in which it can be more effective to play roles built on a few clear elements, but this always limits the wealth of the role's expressible potentialities. Effectiveness must coexist with the variety and the abundance of nuances, expressing the multiform quality of the human experience and therefore opening the possibility of mirroring.

Flexibility vs. rigidity

We have already discussed this point in the section on role constructs, emphasizing that this is the axis on which the creative process pivots, activated by spontaneity. This process allows roles to be modified to suit the relational context, but they also can contain some elements of novelty that cause the transformation of the context itself. Rigid roles produce stuck interactions, where true encounter is unfeasible. The introduction of elements of transformation can be an abrupt event, destroying an equilibrium without anticipating another; or else it can be a dialogical process, in which space and time are given to each system involved to settle in again. The important thing is that the ability to listen is associated with the flexibility, and that we attune ourselves to the other's reactions and answers, so that we can create a dance and not a battle, or, at a higher level of wisdom, turn a battle into a dance.

Engagement vs. disengagement

This structural axis is closely connected with the theme of the distance, of which we have already spoken. Grainger describes its nature using a physical metaphor:

> A role is a potential space which can be moved into by an individual. We can move into that space and fill it with the self, even push its boundaries out to extend and develop the role. On the other hand, we may enter the space tentatively, dipping our toes into it but never filling it with the potentiality of the self.
>
> (Grainger and Duggan 1997: 56)

Distance is the measure of emotional involvement and the regulation of it. The good actor owns an intimate control of the distance and the ability to balance emotional adhesion and separation. Life is not often like this. Landy (1993), taking as a starting point the theories of role in Theodore Sarbin's social psychology and in Thomas Scheff's catharsis theory, calls these polarities:

> 1. 'Overdistance', similar to Sarbin's *noninvolvement*, is characterized by a minimal degree of affect and a maximum degree of rational thought that removes one from one's own feelings and from those of others.
> 2. 'Underdistance', similar to histrionic neurosis, is marked by an overabundance of feeling that floods one's objectivity and reflective capacities.
>
> (Landy 1993: 25)

To these extreme polarities Landy opposes a third possibility (once more a *Middle Course*), which he calls, according to Scheff, *Aesthetic Distance*:

> 'Aesthetic Distance', similar to engrossed acting, is notable for a balance of affect and cognition, wherein both feeling and reflection are available.
>
> (ibid.)

Aesthetic Distance is the meeting point of heart and mind, the place where emotional intelligence is unfolded (see Goleman 1995), where the ability to stay within the emotion and the ability to observe it are melted in the creative gesture, only allowing the controlled flowing of the chaos, the synthesis of Apollo and Dionysus, which is the basic symbolic construction of dramatic art itself.

This point of balance is neither fixed once and for all nor valid in all the person/role interactions; it is different from person to person and from role to role, and it can change along with the context. It is nevertheless possible to develop the faculty to recognize it in different circumstances: this faculty is both a form of sensibility and intuition, and a second level awareness (the awareness to be aware). As Landy points out, the great characters of the theatre are portrayed as very distant from balance: imprisoned by their passions up to insanity or death, or detached and cold calculating people. For action to be, there must be an imbalance, just as a passage of energy can take place only between opposite polarities. 'Without contrary there is no progress,' wrote William Blake. Also in life sometimes it becomes necessary, for building up the individual destiny, to stand in one of the extreme positions, to submit oneself to the emotions' flow by surrendering to them, or to draw oneself out and to act only in name of a rational principle, or at least something looking like it to our eyes. But to remain stuck in one of these two positions or to swing briskly from one to the other is indicative of pathology.

Dramatherapy allows us to experiment with the different possibilities of distance, through progressive shifting along the axis, to find a point of balance: experimentation that is viable also in regard to the other polarities listed. In the 'world' founded by dramatic reality, various degrees of awareness, complexity and flexibility can be experimented with, so we can learn to recognize the signals of the right balance when they come – actually to the point where we learn to play with roles, and therefore also with roles we play in our everyday life in the world, without the risk of harming ourselves or destroying others.

Roles to live by

F is a 30-year-old man. He has had many episodes of hallucination of a persecutory kind. After the death of a mimetically cumbersome father, F did not succeed in managing autonomously in the world anymore, or in creating affective relationships and working projects. He lives in isolation, liable to recurrent moments of thought confusion and crises of anxiety. Among the activities of the day hospital to which he is committed, F takes part in a six-month cycle of Dramatherapy. In the first period, F enacts a set of reassuring roles, based on his world's expectations: he is a reliable Sea Captain, or a Priest taking care of orphans. Of course, the stereotypy of these roles is highlighted by the acting style: predictable, not involved and self-conscious. Once, at about the middle of the run, F was endowed with the role of a Mountain Guide. The trip on the mountains ends with the discovery of a cave where a female wolf is giving birth. F offers to change role and to act as the newborn little wolf. In the following meeting, in an animal game, F chooses the role of the Wolf, an adult wolf this time, that 'kills for the pleasure to kill' and roams free in the forest. The following role, in a scene set in 1000 AD, is the role of the Inquisitor, sending witches to the stake, as well as his own enemies and opponents and, at the very end, even himself. In this role F is more careful, aware of the interaction with the others and therefore more dramatically effective. Above all, he shows a remarkable amount of humour and a greater willingness to play. The following role is again a Sea Captain (F is very keen on the sea), but this time played with a nuance of lightness and a certain sense of relaxation. Only in the next-to-last meeting can F find the words to tell the group of the painful visions he had many years ago during a cruise (a witches' Sabbath electing him as Satan), so that the group can comment empathically upon them.

The roles played by F across the whole process, a small part of which I have mentioned, are containers within which many elements of his experience of the world are joined together. The result of this aggregation is something that both belongs and does not belong to him. It belongs to him in the sense that the imaginative and emotional contents are his own, but the form and the performance modes are bound to the context; they have to be negotiated and set in relationship with the others. The components of these contents are elements of his inner world, at times clear – as they belong to his self image (his own concept of identity) – at times confused and scarcely aware, finding visibility in the role; and mimetic elements, connected with pre-existing forms and expectations. But they are also symbolic elements, whose presence resounds in the shared play, influencing the emotional hue of it. The role of reliable person, so often chosen by F at the beginning, was enough aligned with a Persona of strong fatherly imprint that he had not been able to manage in his personal life – a sort of poor hero missing his task. This aspect was testified to the eyes of the group by F's frequent collapses on various occasions, in moments when he felt confused or distressed. The group, however, shows benevolence to him, actually in virtue of the empathic understanding of those moments of weakness, leading to the inadequacy of F's performances. Such benevolence is translated into personal trust, not in reference to any assignment, but more simply to the capability to be there: for instance, physically not leaving the place in the moments of difficulty, but remaining to watch. On this safe basis, F can play parts of his own inner world, inexpressible if not through a metaphoric mediation. The birth of the wolf is a moment of passage, which is followed by an epiphany of the dark powers through the wild and bloodthirsty animal. At last, a role subversion: F is the Inquisitor, the one who judges and sentences, who will dance in the fire along with his victims (but of course nobody will die, since it's only theatre). The role of the Sea Captain, to which F returns at the end of the process, has a quite different quality in terms of balance, according to the parameters discussed in the previous paragraph – awareness/unawareness; complexity/simplicity; flexibility/rigidity; engagement/disengagement – from the same role in the beginning. What has happened till now is a heritage that influences the ways in which the role is built and expressed. This new captain is not a hero, not even a demon, but a simple human being reacting as he can, able to be wrong but also able to act with big-heartedness toward the others. In the final telling of his own visions, it seems as if F wanted to communicate to us a subtext – one of the possible ones – of his dramatic journey.

The Jungian psychodramatist Giulio Gasca distinguishes, within the sphere of role potentialities that everybody owns, external and internal roles. He defines them as follows:

> As the external roles are the organizers of the perceptions of the external world, the perceptions of the internal world are organized by the internal or intra-personal roles.
>
> (Gasca 1993: 18)

The external roles are mimetically built through the interaction with others, while the internal roles are imaginatively defined, or else they remain at *endocept* level until they find an occasion to be made up in a form (To quote Gasca again: 'all the impulses, stimuli, memories, desires, fragmentary representations, not organized in ways of action toward the surrounding reality nor aimed at the knowledge of it'). In the area of the internal roles, there is the presence of symbolic nucleuses of aggregation, with strong affective density, around which the raw material of the *endocept* is polarized in forms that do not belong to the direct experience of the individual, but pertain to him as he is part of human kind. Gasca, as a good Jungian, is inclined to draw these forms near to those figures that Jung called 'archetypes of the collective unconscious', finding them in myth, in fairytales and in dreams

Landy, in *Persona and Performance* (1993), conducts research into the pre-existing role forms in dramatic literature, from Greek tragedy to nineteenth-century theatre, and identifies some recurrent roles, both typical and archetypal. Landy has compiled an organized inventory, the *Taxonomy of Roles*. A first general division is into *domains* (Somatic, Cognitive, Affective, Social, Spiritual, Aesthetic). Then follows a sub-division into *classifications*. The *Affective domain*, for instance, is divided into two classifications: *moral* and *feeling states*. Within which classification, the roles are listed by *types* and *subtypes*. Landy defines *quality*, *function* and *style* of each role and provides some examples.

In the space of dramatic reality, these structuring forms, whether expressed by figures belonging to humankind's symbolic heritage or culturally transmitted (even by the imagination of great dramatists), find a visible shape in the imaginative roles evoked by the narrative constructions shared by the group, and they are articulated in stage interactions with the other roles. An elderly bank employee, still recovering from a painful divorce coinciding with his retirement, can discover his need for solidarity among men, evoking the hero of the comic strips of his youth, the cowboy hero Tex Willer. A social worker exhausted by *compassion fatigue* can try to rediscover her humorous vein through acting Daniel Pennac's *Mr Malaussène*, professional scapegoat. A teenager son of a drug addict can find a relief from his sense of guilt by staging himself as Simba of Walt Disney's *Lion King*.

But even when the role I play is built upon a pre-existing figure (a character), its manifestation in the relational here and now is influenced by the presence of other roles, internal or external, embryonic or developed, as well as by other endoceptive elements composing the heritage of my potentialities of role. This presence conditions my interpretation/ performance of the role, just as it happens in life:

> The repertoire of our interpretative possibilities is definitely huge. It however depends only partly on us, for the fact is that the roles are constantly reflected in the counter-roles, the mirrors offered by the world. Such repertoire is only partially conscious, because it is also connected with parts of which we don't have full awareness, and because it depends on countless factors of which we cannot clearly know (our biological substratum, the interpretations of the other subjects and objects etc.). There is, however, a psychological reservoir larger than it can appear, if we limit ourselves to observe only what is made actual in the different circumstances, instead of considering also what is potential, although currently not expressed and nevertheless underlying.
>
> (Perussia 2000: 180)

In the imaginative process of Dramatherapy, the mirrors multiply: the 'as if' is the vital nucleus of the poetic inclination, in the sense that Cox and Theilgaard (1987) give to the word *Poiesis*, that is 'calling something into existence that was not there before'. Called into life, evoked and embodied, innumerable roles can be experimented with, enriching our knowledge of the world and of ourselves. We experiment with roles in our relationship with them, along with the tension between what we believe we know and what is expressed despite our will; and in our relationship with the others through them and through the others' roles. But this happens gently, with no judgement or commitment, and we are authorized to transform them or to drop them when they are no longer useful.

Chapter 4

Structures

> Truth dwells in every human heart, and there we must look for it; and
> we have to be guided by the truth as each other sees it.
>
> (M. K. Gandhi, *Ancient as the Mountains*, 1958)

Moreno's invention[1]

As we already mentioned in the Introduction, the first formulation of the
idea of therapeutic group springs from the experience of Moreno. Since
being a student, Moreno practised with groups of people; he worked with
children, prostitutes and First World War refugees in contexts that we
would nowadays call social work, beginning to study the interaction
networks that are active in groups. But the first formulations of the
principle that the group can be a tool to facilitate the processes of change,
clarification and growth typical of psychotherapy came after experiments
in impromptu theatre (Steigreiftheater). The legend tells that the startling
intuition (comparable to Newton's apple or Archimedes's tub) that gave
birth to the practice and, later, to the theoretical modelling of psychodrama, came about with the famous 'case of Barbara'.[2] Reflecting upon
this episode, Moreno was the first to consider deeply the transformative
flows between life and theatre, between dramatic reality and everyday
reality. It is known that Moreno, after many experiments and changes,
got to a model of psychodrama that he defined as *confessional*, in which
a protagonist is encouraged to expose 'with frankness' his/her own
problems and to stage them. In this formulation, Moreno goes far beyond
the first intuition, in which the process of transformation is triggered
by the relationship with an imaginative role, and he draws near to the
abreaction method of early psychoanalysis, a discipline he had previously

considered with some distrust. The concept of *abreaction* is very similar to Moreno's concept of catharsis; both include the sense of a liberating emotional release.

Putting these phenomena at the core of a therapeutic process leaves open a few questions. A cathartic moment is intensely involving: the flow of the emotions crosses physical bodies, shaking them, and may allow new understandings. But how can we be sure that catharsis leads to a new equilibrium of the person, rather than to an increasing chain of unbalance or, even worse, to a defensive rearranging in an obsolete position? Psychoanalysis has answered by putting this concept in a lower position and conferring the main therapeutic function to other factors (first of all the transference process, therefore affirming the centrality of relationship in healing). In psychodrama such a revising process has not happened and catharsis has remained as an unchallenged queen in the therapeutic field. As a matter of fact, this concept is easy to define and to circumscribe, as it is logically structured on cause/effect categories and connected with objective physical elements. It is, in some sense, more 'palatable' of the more elusive (but probably more stimulating) concepts of *spontaneity* and *tele*.[3] It is also perhaps more 'saleable', as shown by some second-rate psychodrama applications, focused on using catharsis as a 'special effect' aimed at *épater les bourgeois*.

Moreno's model is topologically mirrored in the theatre structure conceived by him and built in Beacon, USA, where the places for actors, audience and director are rigidly separate (see Moreno 1946), and audience has mostly the function of a witness. In psychodrama sessions, a person from the audience can change role and become a protagonist, supported by a company of trained actors providing what Moreno calls *Auxiliary Egos*. But until he gets up and leaves his seat in the stalls, he remains a member of the audience, experiencing a vicarious catharsis (as theorized by Aristotle for the spectators of tragedy). Moreno realized the immense potentiality of the group as a transformation agent, and this intuition brought him to a healing approach that nowadays we would call holistic.[4] But the structuring of psychodrama in therapeutic technique led Moreno to the tripartition of actors/audience/director, which lies at the basis of traditional theatre (and differs from it only as far as dramaturgy is regarded); though he condemned it when he was young (in the same years of Artaud's cry) and called for a theatrical revolution, founded upon improvisation (see Moreno 1923).

The fact is that Moreno ignored the important innovations in regard to the sense of the group brought about by what we called the 'new dramatic paradigm': on the one hand, through a tension towards Artaud's utopia, with the incoming transfer to the group of the totality of the creative dramatic process; on the other, with the recovery of the ritual dimension in its deep meaning of human community foundation. In this view, the group is first of all a creative project. The potential energy of every individual meets the energy of the others, and it grows actual in the creation of shared forms. A feeling of sharing endures under this aesthetical process, expressed in an intense mutual receptivity.

Sue Jennings (1988) reflects upon the fact that a *fil rouge* connects the group experimentations of the theatrical avant-garde of the second half of the nineteenth century with the flowering of the most disparate theories and techniques of group therapies and with, I would add, the increasing interest of sociology in the group as a first organizer of society. Between the accent set on the individual and his/her multifaceted inner world and the worried attention towards mass society and its aberrations, the necessity to consider an intermediary level emerges, the level of face-to-face relationships. The concept of group becomes an explicatory model both for the making of personal identity through meaningful interactions with the others, and for the intimate structures of the community and the relational dynamics supporting it. The resulting hypothesis is that an artificially built group is able, *in certain conditions*, to become a place of experimentation and discovery both of the mimetic/relational fabric that supports (or we'd rather say *makes up*) the individual identity, and of its social dispositions. Not only does every member of the group take, through direct interaction with the others, the function of transformation agent, but the group itself is produced as an entity qualitatively different from the sum of its components, a living organism possessing those characteristics that Bateson (1979) ascribes to 'mind' (intending with this term an aggregate of phenomena that, to be understood, needs 'explanations of a different kind from those enough to explain the characteristics of its constituent parts').

Theatrical community

The conditions within which these potentialities of the group are supposed to grow and bear fruit are the markings of differences between the various theoretical models and group practices of the last decades. Dramatherapy's idea of group is rooted in this general thought, and it founds the conditions for the realization of the group's transformative potential on its own being dramatic art.

Irvin Yalom, in his famous text *Theory and Practice of Group Psychotherapy* (1970), written in the time of greatest diffusion of group practices, in therapy as well as in other fields, states some categories within which the manifold therapeutic factors of the group can be classified, apart from the different theoretical orientations.[5] It can be observed that the therapeutic purpose (the conscious aim of leading the process towards adjustment of the person in their relationships with the world) is not strictly necessary. Many factors of this kind can be found in spontaneous groups, or in groups built upon a task, such as theatre groups. In these, as in Dramatherapy, the direct expression of the transformative factors is tightly connected with the process of group construction as theatrical community. Of course, in a theatre group, even if it is led with sensibility and attention, the aesthetic (productive) task may not match with the therapeutic potentiality or it may collide with it. The two needs can also mingle, creating hybrids that do a good turn neither to theatre nor to therapy. Dramatherapy regards as less important the productive demand, and focuses upon the dramatic process as a drive to change, stressing the therapist's responsibility as a catalyst and guide of group creative process (as we will see in more detail later).

But going back to the therapeutic functions, I shall try to analyse the specific declinations of some of them inside a group conceived as a theatrical community, beginning from what Yalom calls *development of socialization techniques*. We have already synthetically discussed play as experimentation with the world of relationship. In developmental terms, play is the first experience of interpersonal relationships beyond the entourage of primary bonds: it is for the child the first socialization training. The foundation of a play frame, as a point of departure of the dramatic process, suggests this meaning of play: an area of interaction governed by rules which guarantee to everybody the possibility to participate and the freedom to maintain their own vital spaces. Through play, not only does the foundation of the group as interaction area proceed, but also the beginning of the construction of an aesthetical language, peculiar to this group and to no other, which strengthens the cohesion of the group as theatrical community and the sense of belonging. The actor's training in Dramatherapy hinges upon games: we must be especially grateful to Viola Spolin's work for the insight that the actor's job can usefully be turned into game.[6] Her *theatre games* are actions aimed at solving a problem, put to a single person or to the whole group, which demand a level of collaboration. But, Spolin warns, the fact that the solution is not univocal and that endless solutions, all of them correct, are possible, and accordingly the absence of approval or disapproval from the leader, suggesting a more general suspension of the judgement, reduces the competitiveness and opens the way to collaboration:

This combination of individuals mutually focussing and mutually involved creates a true relation, a sharing of a fresh experience. Here old frames of reference topple over as the new structure (growth) pushes its way upwards, allowing freedom of individual response and contributions. Individual energy is released, trust is generated, inspiration and creativity appear as all the players play the game and solve the problem together. 'Sparks' fly between people when this happens.

(Spolin 1963: 24)

The 'sparks' Spolin speaks of are lightings of empathy: the immediate (pre-reflexive) experience of listening and of mutual support. An exercise I often use in various types of group is an elaboration of a theatre game invented by Keith Johnstone (1979). Standing in circle, each member of the group in turn addresses the right-side companion, and leads him/her at the centre, delivering to him/her an imaginary gift.[7] The other will unwrap it and show it to the group, declaring what it is. The problem that I have to solve, in the role of receiver, is to think of an object and to mime its use; in the role of the giver it is to put the other at ease, helping them in the assignment. Of course, the most relevant dramatic work for me is on receiver's role, and it is crucial for me to feel a non-judging sharing by the others, the permission to give a solution that is personally mine, even if it is not remarkably 'original' or 'creative'. Whether it is a book, a succulent plant, a pup or a spaceship, what is important is that it is here, imaginatively in front of us. If the audience is willing to believe – and the audience is made by each of us – the very action of the game, the tiny performance, becomes a gift for the group. But I also have the chance to be the ambassador of the authorization by the group, entering onstage as a 'stooge', allowing the action to start and sustaining the protagonist in accomplishing his task.

This is a delicate role. I have to facilitate the other's work without invading it, to help others to express themselves, while avoiding over-lapping them. If I place my personal objectives before the purpose of the game, trying to show my originality or my actor's cleverness, for instance, the game simply doesn't work. I remember a young educator in a training group. She had studied theatre and she was eager to show it so she entered the stage miming the dragging of a heavy load, and shaping the outlines of an enormous, half-spherical object (she declared later she had thought about a pumpkin), embarrassing the person that received it, who had to try hard to guess what it was. The circuit of the gifts was interrupted, and with it the very possibility of the group to authorize itself as affective container. But what usually happens is that the metaphoric content of the game, with its ritual components, produces an atmosphere of benevolence: exchanging symbolic gifts in the space of 'as if' embodies the sense of cooperation in the here and now of the dramatic process, and it strengthens the relational principle of altruism, the mutual concession of the 'permission to exist'. The bond of mutual influencing between the 'world' and the world is mediated by the world of the group, a microcosm that mirrors the macrocosm, but which is also the place where the possibilities of reinventing the world through the invention of the 'world' are unfolded. As agent of connection between 'reality' and 'imagination', the Dramatherapy group is a transitional space, in which everyone is granted permission to re-elaborate the conflicting knots of their own relationship with the world, reconstruing them imaginatively. The gesture on stage recalls a fragment of the world of the person performing it, but as it is not an imitation but a creation, it becomes universal, speaking not only of me and you and him and her, but of all of us, as we are part of the same kind and the same adventure.

Affects and images

The 'embrace game'[8] is an exercise I often use in the first phases of a training group. Being an exercise that implies a powerful physical contact, it is to be used with care. With teenager groups, for instance, in which Eros's urges are on perpetual alert, the physical contact can be embarrassing because spoiled by a sexual interpretation. In groups of people suffering from mental disorders, in which the emotional sensitivity is in a tottering equilibrium, the embrace can emotionally be felt as an unbearable invasion. In such situations, it is preferable to think of this exercise more as a goal than as a starting point. I would like to describe it, however, because I think it can be a useful analogy to reflect upon the group in the dramatic process.

The exercise is divided into three phases. At the beginning, the participants stand in a circle. This is already the first task of the group: holding each other's hands, they can make some attempts to find a circular shape that satisfies everybody. Given their simplicity, these attempts do not need to be guided, nor to involve any verbal exchange. The sense of cooperation begins with a simple spatial operation, and a first physical contact is established. Besides, the circle allows everybody to be seen by the others, but nobody, for the moment, is the centre of attention. The therapist explains the rules, which are very simple. At the agreed signal, a person (*A*) moves from his/her position and goes and embraces the person to the left (*B*), who gives back the embrace. After a little while, the embrace loosens and *A* embraces the person at *B*'s left (*C*). *A* continues and embraces *D*, while *B* moves and embraces *C*. Then *A* embraces *E*, while *B* embraces *D*, and so on, until everybody returns to their former place. At the end of the cycle, everybody has twice embraced all the others: once giving and once receiving. If the game is proposed during the first meeting, when the group members are not yet acquainted with each other, usually the therapist 'rolls the ball', so taking the role of example and guarantor of the rules (as well as providing the rhythm of the exercise).

Is it a real or a metaphoric embrace? Of course, it misses the motivation of a real embrace: it is strange to find ourselves embracing a stranger or a person with whom we have nothing but formal relationships. But the very gesture of the bodily contact, of feeling the holding and the breath of the other, of perceiving the reciprocity of the action, is the mimetic vehicle of an unfocused emotional state. It is the routine of the game, its choreographic construction, that provides the frame, the proper distance to live the emotion; mimetically reconstructing it inside us, but also upholding the correct separation. The emotion is expressed at first in light embarrassment; giggles and accents of surprise are heard, then laughter turns into smiles, and a pleasant feeling of encounter spreads in the group. The affective temperature of the group rises because everybody has the chance to approach the other in a situation that, though contrived, exalts mimetic exchanges.

The second phase of the exercise has the same structure as the previous one, but with a different connotation. Here an acknowledged point of view of 'as if' is brought in. The therapist asks everyone to put their head, in the stance of looking for comfort, on their companion's shoulder, who will welcome him/her in their arms and comfort him/her for a while. In comparison with the previous phase, there are two meaningful differences. First, people are asked for a deliberate pretending: a level of fiction mediates a behaviour that, as in the first part, involves close contact. Second, the positions are no longer symmetrical but complementary, and an inversion of role occurs, so that each one is allowed to take on the role of the other. The contact is more intimate, as it is mimetically related to more immediately acknowledgeable situations, and therefore puts into action what Stanislavskij called 'emotional memory'. However, the distance is greater because the meta-communication frame is clearer, not only suggested by the structure of the exercise, but also by its content. The declared pretence sets us free to live the positive feelings evoked by being welcome and sustained, and the joy of giving in comforting the other without being wholly involved. Along with this, there grows the feeling that the group is a place in which the emotional flows can be experienced without fear.

The third phase keeps the same cyclical scheme, but this time the instructions are to let oneself fall into the other's arms; the other will support you and again put you in a position to fall once more on the next companion. There is also an inversion of roles, underlining the mutual responsibility: I support you, so later you will support me. Even here the 'as if' is explicit, but with a further difference. While in the previous phase the narrative frame containing the gesture is connected to a real possibility in the world (therefore related to actual relational experiences), here it illustrates a metaphor. This metaphor reminds us of a dimension of the relationship – the act of relying on someone else – that cannot be reduced to an exemplifying action, but is concerning the whole symbolic horizon of the turning toward the other. In this sense, it is a gesture more abstract than the ones above, as it is not similar to any real gesture in the world, except perhaps the flight of children into their parents' arms, or being supported in a fainting fit. In a certain sense, it shares the meaning of both: of the former, the presence of both fear and trust in the child's action (Sue Jennings calls it the *risk/safety paradigm*) and the playfulness of parents grabbing them; of the latter, the feeling of losing oneself – the emerging of our own frailty and need – and of helping and sustaining the other. But the sense of the metaphor goes beyond these suggestions and straight to the heart of the relationship itself: trusting the other 'because yourself'.

The construction of the group as a theatrical community begins from the here and now of the physical presence of people, in their being originally body-selves. The body in action stirs the mimetic flows, which allow me to accept the other as similar in the core fact of being a body. Although this body can be different from mine, contracted, flabby, limited in functions and expressions, in the meeting and in the contact deep analogies are disclosed, and I realize that differences are at a quantitative rather than qualitative level. But my coming into play as a body is connected also with the activation of an emotional sphere, vague and nonthematic, which meets the other's sphere, producing a sort of indistinct emotional aura that nevertheless defines the group as a special space. It is as if a potential emotional energy is freed, waiting to be channelled. This image reminds me of Bateson's 'third criterion of the mental process' (1979): 'The mental process needs a collateral energy.' Does it exist something like a 'psychic energy'? Actually, binding this concept to the models of physical sciences (of *Pleroma* rather than of *Creatura*, to quote Bateson again glossing Plato), leads to blind alleys: whether this happens by reconnecting it to the area of bodily energy, as in Reich's *orgonic* theory; or comparing it to some 'strange' aspects of physics' advanced models, as in the curious but fascinating Arthur Koestler's conjecture (1972), hypothesizing the existence of 'mental particles', comparable to the *neutrins* of subatomic physics. The fact is that the concept of energy includes its being quantifiable. Therefore it is not applicable to phenomena that cannot be measured. Our Western languages do not have terms to describe these kinds of things (unlike the non-European languages, which have an infinity of words with a profusion of shades: from Polynesian *mana*, to Indian *tejas*, to Chinese *li*). Perhaps the only terminology that is at our disposal in the Western world pertains to religious experience, from which the disciplines professing a scientific study of human things turn away with disdain (except in rare exceptions). Grainger, using some elements of the Christian tradition to describe the sense of the group in Dramatherapy, adopts the term love:

> It is the love which bestows and receives gifts. The satisfaction it receives is that of giving in order to create relationship; it receives as part of the gift. This love of exchanging beings is sociogenic. It is experienced as originating elsewhere, because it moves backwards and forwards among people, forging invisible ties among everywhere it touches. Christian tradition calls it agape, and distinguishes it from eros, whose aim is to enlarge the self by direct enjoyment of the other.
>
> (1995: 14)

From another point of view, we could describe this group energy as a tension toward a mutual influencing, yielding some changes that, qualitatively and quantitatively, cannot even be imagined in loneliness. In the Dramatherapy process, this tension is addressed toward a creative remixing of the equilibrium among the components of the individual identity: consciousness, body and roles. Triggered by the imaginative action, this remixing can lead to a new, more comprehensive balance. Through the mediation of the 'as if', I can focus on universal images that become actual in the here and now of the relationship, entering the imaginative heritage of each and every person. The first image is the image of care, which reminds us of the primary experience (ontogenetic and phylogenetic) of nutrition and nurturing, developing – in relational terms – trust and confidence, benevolence and not-judging acceptance. Upon these bases, the group builds its own access to the territory of the metaphor, in a double sense. Images, words, roles and stories, created and shared in group, tell about life and show the world in the 'world.' But meanwhile, the group itself, in its creative effort, revealing the strength and the weakness of each one without judging, is metaphor of the greatness and the frailty of human nature.

This character of the group as a community of people that meets to create what Bateson called 'its own metaphor' founds the possibility of empathy. Empathy is not to be intended as identification in the other, but rather, as Edith Stein maintained, expanding our experience to include the other:

> [According to Edith Stein, empathy is] to widen our own experience, to be able to welcome other people's pain and joy, maintaining the distinction between me and the other. Empathy is 'to realize', to catch the reality of others' pain and joy, not to suffer or to rejoice in first person or identify ourselves with the other. [. . .] Empathy attests therefore the possibility of the circulation or communication of the experience, not because two subjects become one, melt or find an analogy and a mysterious identity, but because it is possible to refer to something that is not me, but it is not a thing, it is the lived reality of another human being.
>
> (Boella and Buttarelli 2000: 69–70)

PROCESS

> True poetry is the *arcanum* that connects us to life, that separates us from life. Separating – only by separating can we really live – if we separate, even death is bearable, only what is mixed is horrible [. . .] – but just as separating is essential, so is connecting – the *aurea catena Homeri*.
>
> (Hugo von Hofmannsthal, *Andrew or The Reunited*, 1932, fragments)

Ritual and drama

The hero's journey, we have already mentioned, is the *monomyth* of the transformation, the change-telling narrative structure, pointing to the very sense of becoming. All the stories about the passage from one existence level to another, including even our own life stories, echo it. In religious myths, the change is often marked by death and transfiguration of the hero, born to a new life in the sap of his people. In fairytales, the return is often related to a status change and to the achievement of wisdom and wealth. But stories, all the stories, illustrate a deep truth of the human condition: that the course of existence is mutation, and that mutation cannot be attained without danger. Difficulties, accidents and obstacles can occur, but it is actually in facing them and overcoming them, in the act of going beyond and transcending, and in the effort and pain of the struggle, that we are led to a new, deeper awareness of the sense of our own journey.

In essence, the narrative structure of the hero's journey can be divided into three phases: the preparation (including the call and the departure); the actual journey (with the trials, the battles and the fulfilments); the return (with the recognition of the transformations occurred and the resulting renewal of the community). This tripartite structure of the hero's journey is comparable with the phases of the ritual process studied by Van Gennep: he defines them as *pre-liminal*, *liminal* and *post-liminal* (from *limen*, threshold). The first phase pivots on the *construction of the present*: the bonds with the past are cut off and the participants are immersed in an unconditioned now, in which the collective power to go toward the future is evoked:

> Thus the rite prepares and enables us for the future by disarming the past. Not all past time, but our own past in its negative aspect, which drains the present of its meaning and significance. The rite allows us to understand in the present and live in the present.
>
> (Grainger 1974: 113)

In the *pre-liminal* phase, the participants take off their old clothes and get ready to face the new, purifying and strengthening themselves in body and spirit.

The *liminal* phase is when time has a stop: it is the time-without-time of the 'germination and preparation for the new birth' (ibid.: 116). If the metaphor of the previous phase is the grave (the symbolic death marking the removal of ways of being and meanings of the past), the metaphor of this phase is the womb (the hidden and protected place where new life takes shape). Indeed, it is the time of chaos and uncertainty, in which we are asked to look our own fears right in the eye and to recognize our own limits and vulnerability in the presence of the absolute Otherness. But it is also the time when wisdom of humankind enters us through the stories of those that before us, and for us, have faced the distress and pain of the passage and the shining of the encounter.

In the third phase (*post-liminal*) time again starts its course, but it is a renewed time (ibid.: 119). It is the time in which we celebrate the new life that has entered and regenerated us. The Encounter gives light to the meeting with the others, with those people who have taken part in the rite and who have shared with us the joy and grief of the journey, conferring on it a new value, the value of the refounding of the community as part of a greater destiny, which surrounds it and justifies it.

Even if, as Grainger notices, there is a shared ground between the dramatic and the ritual processes, there are also remarkable differences:

> The theatre does not have to concern itself with the proclamation of a religious message; the parts played are those of members of human social groups, human beings not gods nor a mixture of the two categories. The audience's involvement is understood to be optional rather than in any sense compulsory for the attainment of authentic human-ness. Most important of all, the focus of encounter is between human beings rather than human being and divinity.
>
> (Grainger and Duggan 1997: 62)

Richard Schechner has devoted his whole life to studying from a unique, inclusive conceptual point of view what he calls 'performance activity', in which he includes, besides theatre and religious rituals, sports, games, the social and institutional rites and the performances of everyday life.[9] According to Schechner, ritual and theatre embody the opposite fundamental polarities in regard to the purposes of the performance, which he identifies in 'effectiveness' and 'entertainment'. In Figure 4.1 we see how these polarities are expressed in ritual and in theatre.

The dramatic process in Dramatherapy stands in a midpoint position between the two polarities (once more, a middle course), sharing features of both. It is worthwhile analysing some aspects of this statement. Ritual is an action aiming at a change; so is Dramatherapy. Dramatherapy's objectives are clearly defined: first of all the improvement of people's self-identity, with the expansion, both in a quantitative and qualitative sense, of the repertoire of available roles, along with the growth of imagination, interpersonal abilities and communication. But the work aimed at achieving the change enfolds in a gentle way, fundamentally cheerful and playful, without sweat and tears. Dramatherapy time is also a time of fun, of enjoyment with the others. Indeed, there is room for tensions and sufferings, but they are welcomed with warmth and benevolence. They are never refused or denied, but envisaged as human experiences which can be shared. This vision is not within the frame of a theology that looks at an Other as a source of sense and authorization, but finds in the person near me, in the playmate who is like me and with me – meat, blood and word – even if other than me, the incarnation of a

EFFECTIVENESS	ENTERTAINMENT
Ritual	**Theatre**
Results.	Fun.
Bond with an absent Other.	Only the people present.
Symbolic time.	Emphasis on the here and now.
Performers are possessed,	Performers are aware
in trance.	of what they do.
The audience participates.	The audience observes.
The audience believes.	The audience judges.
Criticism is discouraged.	Criticism is supported.
Collective creativity.	Individual creativity.

Figure 4.1 The polarity effectiveness/entertainment according to Richard Schechner (1988, adapted from Deriu 1999)

feeling of communion, connecting me with you and him and her, and all of us with the whole world of people and things that we can create together (the dimension of universality that Yalom sets among the principal therapeutic factors). Dramatherapy is a form of dramatic art that, even if not explicitly religious or based on beliefs systems, has nonetheless a potential spiritual quality similar to that of ritual.

The dramatic cycle

In its essential structure, the dramatic process of Dramatherapy has more analogies with the ritual cycle (with the due differences stated before) than with the theatre. Like the ritual, the process develops in three phases that I have called *Foundation, Creation* and *Sharing* (Pitruzzella 2000). Every phase generates a flow of unbalancing and rebalancing, taking a different point of departure (which is also a point of view) in every phase. The *Foundation* phase starts from the body. Roles and stories are the protagonists of the *Creation*. The individual's consciousness, their provisional 'I', reappears transformed in the *Sharing* phase. The dramatic cycle risks the presuppositions of the individual identity, recomposing them in new possible conformations through an interpersonal experience:

It is this three-fold configuration that communicates a sense of completeness, of something real having happened, a genuine event which has changed the nature of the reality as real events must inevitably do in order to be real.

(Grainger 1995: 9)

I will try now concisely to describe these three phases.

Foundation phase

The Foundation phase starts when the first agreement is made. It can be preceded by some individual meetings with each of the participants, in which expectations are clarified, the possible objectives of the process are arranged to the individual needs, rules and limits are established. These meetings can be useful for the therapist to get information on the personal stories of the participants, told from their own point of view.[10] When individual meetings are not feasible, or when the Dramatherapy group is already included in a therapeutic project (for instance when it is part of the activities of a psychiatric day hospital or therapeutic community), then the contract explaining the ground rules and possible objectives must be made collectively during the first meetings. This is a rather delicate operation for various reasons. The word 'theatre' may provoke restlessness. It can evoke the uneasiness to perform under the others' judging eyes. The experience 'to be another', even in a defined place and time, can be associated with fear of loss of one's own identity, rather than with the chance to find it out. Alternatively, expectations can be aroused 'to be an actor', not only in the sense 'to learn the trade' but also in the sense of an identification with a desirable professional role, a status and an identity imagined as a goal to be achieved (while actually the actor's life is in general far from happy). It is therefore necessary to give a cosy and reassuring message, discouraging any misunderstandings.

Another aspect to consider is the fact that theatre does not necessarily belong to the cultural universe of the participants. More than once I had to deal with people who had never been in a theatre and for whom the only available reference was the all-pervading television. In these cases, the idea itself of drama must be created little by little. These are often very interesting experiences in which the dramatic language must be built upon the basic expressive abilities of the subjects involved, and therefore directly from their world of interpretation/performance, which must come into contact with that of the others. This encounter demands creative solutions, not conditioned by preset styles or techniques, especially when different communication modes meet (as with people belonging to different social or ethnic contexts). The encounter is possible because, in the Foundation phase, the body speaks more than anything else. The body playing, in this phase, is both an approaching means, a vehicle of an emotional activation through an immediately available medium, and a factor of separation. In the frame of play, *my* body is just *a* body, a simple tool of the game, through which I am allowed to take part in the meeting without the need to disclose myself too much. My 'true' self can be hidden, for the moment. The body here is both primal experience and mask, and it is the point of departure for the construction of a shared dramatic language.

This phase is also a phase of training, in which spontaneity and narrative ability are practised, and the access to the 'as if' dimension is prepared; the dimension that is at the core of the second phase, the Creation.

Creation phase

In the Creation phase, the imaginative worlds come together and mould each other, embodying in the dramatic reality. The work of art that is created is temporary and provisional (impermanent, Buddhists would say), but it is nonetheless real, a creative action that produces a visible and meaningful form. In this phase stories and scenes are born, the role constructs take shape and become actual in the interaction. If the process is developed in a harmonious way, with the correct balance between tension and distance, between collective and individual creativity (see Schechner's model quoted before), the actions 'flow naturally, like the steps of a dance, so that the dramatic action maintains its impetus and meaning' (Grainger and Duggan 1997: 127).

In this Creation phase, I can live the dramatic space as a place devoted to me, at my disposal to populate with materials to transform. I will try to clarify this aspect with a story. G is a 13-year-old boy from Albania. Abandoned in his earliest youth by his parents together with his little sister, he has spent part of his short life in an orphanage (and the quality of that experience is witnessed by the fact that G has a finger gnawed by mice). At the age of five, he is given in adoption to a Sicilian couple (who, to tell the truth, would have preferred to take up only his little sister) and brought to a small town near Palermo. The new parents are people of poor culture and scarce affective consistency, with few resources to heal the wounds of G, who gives more and more vent to his restlessness with incomprehensible and uncontrollable behaviours: destructive and self-harming crises, repeated escapes and very dangerous deeds. G has been attending the centre for almost one and a half years and, little by little, he is learning to know himself and to have relationships. We are at the last meeting before the summer vacations. Although we are near the sea, the heat is very intense and many people – both workers and clients – are already on holiday. In the youngest group (13 to 15 years) there are only four of us: M (a colleague psychologist in the youth psychiatric unit), E, a 13-year-old girl with a slight learning disability, which has given rise to a serious personality disorder, G, and me. The last meeting before a long break is always very difficult and I imagine it must be even more for G, who has lived on rejections. Even if it is a temporary separation, arranged and prepared with care so that it can be a chance of growth rather than suffering, it is anyway an event that triggers deep feelings, often awkward to think about and tell. Both the kids are craving to begin the workshop. G runs and asks for the keys of the room from the caretaker (who has become a great friend of his) and opens the door. Considering the enthusiasm, I decide to move right away into the dramatic action (the Foundation phase being summed up in the action of taking off our shoes before entering the workshop and a short greeting ritual). I ask the kids if there is anything they feel like staging to say goodbye in this temporary parting. E confusedly tells a dream, where parental figures overlap with her carers, with ambivalent interactions: too hard to disentangle. G proposes to work instead on the plot of a Walt Disney film, whose title is *Escape On All Fours*. The suggestion is enthusiastically accepted: we all remember a masterly enactment of G as the Tramp in *Lady and the Tramp*, a true milestone in the dramatic journey of the group. The story is once more a story of animals. There were once a dog and a cat, bought by a couple in a shop, unbeknown to both. Why? To give a surprise: a Christmas gift. The dog and the cat learn to know each other: at first they are mistrustful, they scowl at each other and quarrel, then, little by little, they even become friends. One sad day, their owners have to leave and they send them to a pets hostel. But the hostel holder, seemingly so kind and smiling, turns out to be a treacherous tyrant, who parts them and abuses them: so the two decide to run away. After many hard times and dangers (among which is an escape from the claws of the dogcatcher), at last they are found by a friend of their owners, who brings them back home.

The roles are instantly assigned: G will be the cat, E the dog, and M and I will play all the other roles, beginning with the owners. Wisely, M adds a hint of distance, suggesting that the owners are not wife and husband but brother and sister, and the play can begin. G plays the role of the cat for the entire time without using words. Every now and then he goes out of role (he stops the game) to give some cue for the sequel, then returns to being a cat and expressing himself in a cat-like way. We witness some dramatic sequences of astonishing bliss: the meeting of the two animals and their mutual acquaintance, with a succession of progressive attempts at approach, in which each other's trustworthiness is tested; the suffering of the imprisonment and the yearning for freedom; the losing and finding themselves. Their coming back home is a moment of great emotion; both G and E surrender to physical contact, rubbing themselves and asking for cuddles. G is outstandingly relaxed. His physical tone is different from usual when, even in an embrace, elements of aggressiveness and fear are shown. At the end of the meeting, after a snack taken together with all the others, G asks me to help him make a kite. This activity was, nearly one year ago, my first true opportunity to encounter him (at the beginning G did not succeed in tolerating the group for more than 10 or 15 minutes). We make a red kite with an orange tail, flying high in the sky, and G asks me if he can take it home. That delicate object of coloured paper, which flies with the wind and then comes back, is the witness of our being together, waiting for meeting again. With his story, and with his living presence in it, G has given us a synthesis of his feelings and of his efforts to face them, inviting us to enter them, asking for reassurance and confirmations that can pass only through the nonthematic language of the body, which expands in an imaginative sphere that authorizes, surprises and cradles us.

This suspended moment in which four people crouch on a carpet, exchanging cuddles, is a *state of grace*,[11] in which all the meanings are transcended and reconnected in a symbolic unity that speaks for itself, an experience that does not need any other explanations. When moments of this kind occur, it is not necessary to emphasize them: all the people recognize the extent of them and everybody is deeply affected by them. Immediate comments are not often possible (except at times a generic 'it has been so nice!'). Nevertheless, the whole group perceives them as crucial moments in which the group rises and turns into nourishment.

These may be moments of great emotion, in which tears might flow, or of great hilarity. I cherish a memory, for instance, of a scene in a training group that was almost halfway through its run. The exercise from which the scene developed is the 'mirror sculpt' game (a variation of the sculpture games broadly used in actors' training, which are at the core of the 'Boal method'). A subgroup quickly sets up a position, creating an unintentional human sculpture. The other subgroup observes and then forms the same figure, to which they will give a meaning, through the improvisation of both verbal and nonverbal interactions. One of the subgroups creates a curious and somewhat anxious figure. Four people lie flat on their backs, star shaped, with the tops of their heads touching; they have arms and legs flexed upward. At first sight, it reminds me of a four-mirrored version of Kafka's nightmare. The actors, however, after some efforts, decide that what they are doing is holding up a weight with arms and legs. 'Come on, hold it!' 'It's so heavy!' 'Come on, we can make it!' Little by little we understand that the thing they are trying to move is a closet, an enormous closet that overhangs them and could crush them. From that unhappy position, there are serious doubts that the manoeuvre can succeed. The tension grows more and more, with intense shouts that increase up to paroxysm, along with the increasing difficulty to resolve the situation. At the point of maximum effort, there is a sort of explosion and a person squirts out, rolling. There is no more closet, there are no more cries, there is only a great silence. She, alone, in the centre of the stage, after an endless moment of perplexity, utters a wail as a newborn child. At this point, everybody, audience and actors, bursts with laughter and there is a thunder of applause. The metaphor that had been created was freeing and of good omen, and it marked a turning point in a training process that had been fatiguing and uncertain, but of which we started to glimpse the ultimate sense.

Sharing phase

The third phase of the dramatic cycle is the Sharing. This is the phase of exit, in which the group returns to everyday consciousness crossing back the border of the dramatic reality:

> The group celebrates the end of their own journey, going again along the stages and sharing the contents, beginning from their own lived experiences. An evaluation and a critical re-examination of the scenes go along with such emotional exchange, starting with the reflection on their effectiveness as communications. In the *Sharing*, the group becomes established as affective container and is validated as a place in which it is possible to explore conflicts and give voice, on stage, to repressed emotions and shadowy parts of themselves.
>
> (Pitruzzella 1998: 9)

Often verbal comments are useful but they are not always necessary. The awareness of the journey is present here and it can be expressed in symbolic and imaginative terms – with a gesture or a sign, or even in verses, or simply by keeping quiet and being there.

The room is again a room of the world, with a door that separates us from it and puts us in contact with it, and that can be crossed through, bringing with us an extra experience. Greeting each other, we make an appointment for the next meeting.

THERAPIST

> The first and only juggler, and I must be the best,
> I love to see the rings spin, never at rest,
> Up in the air, and back to me:
> What it will do, I just can't see.
> (Robin Williamson, *Juggler's Song*)

Keeping the fire alight

In *Demian*, his great *bildungsroman* written in 1917, Hermann Hesse tells us of the meeting of the protagonist, Emil Sinclair, with a bizarre master of life, the organist Pistorius:

> 'Come here,' he called me. 'We will do some practical philosophy: let's keep quiet, lie down on our bellies and think.'
> He struck a match and set the heap of paper and wood on fire. Once aroused the flame, he fed the fire with lovely caution. I went close to him on the worn-out carpet. He stared at the flames that also attracted me, so we remained a long time in front of the crackling fire winding and hissing, lowering and wriggling, quivering and sparkling, finally smouldering under the ashes. 'The adoration of the fire was not the silliest thing people invented,' he muttered.

Only later the young man understands the meaning that the unusual experience had for him:

> The contemplation of such images, the abandonment to irrational, strange and complex forms of the nature, causes in us a sense of agreement among our heart and the wish that gave birth to these forms; suddenly we have the temptation to mistake them for our whims, for our creations; we see the limits between the nature and us tremble and blur, and we begin to know the atmosphere in which we don't know whether the images on the retina are produced from external or internal impressions. Never like in this exercise do we

make the simple and easy discovery that we are creative, than our soul is always part of the continuous creation of the world.

Contemplating the fire, looking at it, as Blake would have said, 'not with the eyes but through the eyes', Emil discovers the creative imagination, that is, the heart of the art that connects us with the world and with the universe. But this contemplation can exist only if there is someone who lights the fire, feeding it 'with lovely caution'. He has to arrange paper and firewood of various sizes: the thin and dry twigs that easily catch fire and generate an intense but fleeting heat; the middle-sized branches, wrist-thick, which guarantee a strong and continuous flame; and finally the logs, that will be enduring nourishment for the fire. He has to make the first spark glow and he must blow, softly or strongly, to sustain the newborn little flame. He has then to watch it and to keep it in balance: to add firewood or to move it to make it burn harder, or to remove the logs to slow it down. Finally, he has to gently let it extinguish, preserving the embers for the next day.

Can I succeed in making both things together, to contemplate and to act? The task is not impossible, but it demands a deep knowledge and great concentration skill. I must learn to master a technique to the point of being able to apply it without thinking too much, and also continually adapting it to suit the situation. I must also learn to maintain a persistent attention while doing another activity. I believe that the dramatherapist is called to a very similar assignment. He has to take care of the kindling of the dramatic process, and to keep it alive, intervening when necessary. At the same time, he has to observe, not only filling it with meanings, but also fully taking part in it, understanding it imaginatively and emotionally. Above all, he has to be able to observe himself meanwhile, which means to correct faults and to learn from experience.

The general function of the therapist in a Dramatherapy process is to promote and to check the conditions in which everybody can use drama as a tool for improving their own well-being. If therapy is service, the dramatherapist is a person who serves the other persons, able to understand their needs, to support them along the way and to help them in difficulties. But in the meantime he serves the dramatic process, aware that only through it, a basically artistic creative process, the change can occur. According to Landy:

> The essential role of the dramatherapist is to embody the creative principle and mirror it, to return it back on the client.
>
> (in Jennings 1992: 110)

The first and most important resource that the dramatherapist has to make available to the people is his/her own creativity: then, imagination and spontaneity, ability to listen to the messages of one's own internal world and aesthetic taste. Even if the studies on creativity from a cognitive point of view are many and meaningful, they cannot exhaust the complexity of the matter.[12] Art, as Nelson Goodman maintains, overcomes the 'tyrannical dichotomy' between the emotional and the cognitive; the individual creative process includes the affective universe of the person. 'We can never be creative people,' stated the Jungian analyst Aldo Carotenuto (1991: 677) 'if we don't allow ourselves to live the affectivity.' Drama-therapists therefore come into play as whole persons, with their emotional intelligence, connected with their being body-selves, dynamic fulcrums of a mimetic net. The bodily awareness that is also self-perception, that is, intuitive responsiveness to the bodily signals connected to emotions, allows gaining access to the empathic experience of the other, even in absence of words. This receptive attitude rules the very possibility of the creative process:

> Receptiveness can be considered a way to go and meet Dionysus and his gifts. Receptiveness can be in fact defined as the attitude that prepares us for the passage.
>
> (Carotenuto 1991: 657)

The passage Carotenuto refers to is the alchemical transmutation of the negative powers that dwell inside the human being, hindering his full development and his potentialities, in positive powers, that nourish and guard him. If we have chosen drama as the medium for this transmutation, then it is necessary that the dramatherapist has the inclination to elaborate what he carefully receives and to give it back in dramatic terms (as stimuli, cues and structures).

In this sense, the work of the dramatherapist is a work of ceaseless translation, of mediation and communication between the world and the 'world'. He is like a stalker, the character of Tarkovskij's film, who guides the travellers in unknown territories, relying on the fact that he knows them because he has already crossed that threshold.

Equipment and luggage

Sue Jennings's Mandala

According to Sue Jennings, the dramatherapist in action must be able to manage four 'internal roles': the patient, the therapist, the supervisor and the creative artist. These roles have:

> to be kept in balance, and constantly nurtured and stimulated. [. . .] The internal patient brings together those aspects of ourselves that have made similar journey to those of our clients and patients. [. . .] The internal therapist brings the whole range of therapeutic knowledge and understanding to bear in the situation. [. . .] The internal supervisor is able to stand a little apart and look in. [. . .] The internal artist informs all the other internal states – patient, therapist and supervisor as well as existing in its own right. It is often the creative impulse that enables the supervisor to help the drama to move on, it assists the therapist in dramatic content and structure, it can connect with the internal patients, especially in despair and find creative ways through the morass.
>
> (Jennings 1990: 47–50)

Jennnings has elaborated her model and synthesized it in a Mandala scheme, as we can see in Figure 4.2. This scheme includes the four 'internal roles' in a larger perspective, concerning the dramatherapist as a whole person. They might be considered therefore as expressions of the basic aspects of individual personality in a specific frame (the professional role).

Jennings puts *Belief* – the system of principles in which we believe, that are the key constructs through which we give meaning to the world – at the heart of the Mandala. Faith, beliefs and values are not seen as superstructures or sublimations, but as a rooting in the world's breeding ground, a spiritual core that moulds and influences all the other parts. 'The Faith of a Dramatherapist' is the subtitle of one of the most enlightening texts by Roger Grainger (1995), which focuses on the fact that attention to the spiritual aspects of existence is a constant of the dramatherapist's vocation. Grainger exposes the results of a research that utilizes Kelly's Repertory Grid Test upon a sample of practitioners, to notice the presence of spiritual elements in the conception they have of their own job. The valuable datum emerging is that the presence of implicit religious constructs is at a rate of 49 to 110 and their importance as connected with the other constructs is far greater than constructs of other kinds. In other words, Grainger writes:

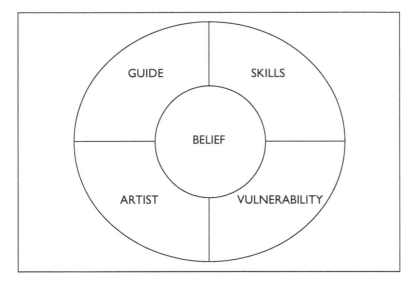

Figure 4.2 Sue Jennings's *Mandala* (from: Jennings 1998: 124)

There were almost as many 'religious' factors in the dramatherapist's way of looking at Dramatherapy as there were factors of other kind; and they were structurally more important in contributing to the way that the individuals in the group organised their awareness, including as they did attitudes, ideas and experiences of considerable importance for their own personal interpretation of life.

(Grainger 1995: 114)

It is however important to underline that the constructs indicated as implicitly religious are not related to specific faiths but have a rather general spiritual connotation. Included in this category are constructs involving:

(a) the relationship between and among persons, love and under-standing; (b) morality and personal responsibility; (c) the use of imagery to express awareness of what is reached out but not grasped; (d) a sense of human destiny and purpose; the transcendence of present experience.

(ibid.: 114)

On the other hand, if we return to Yalom's list of therapeutic factors, we notice that at least three of them have a connotation that we might consider to be implicitly religious: *Infusion of hope, Universality, Altruism*. As for me, I would gladly put as an epigraph in the middle of my personal Mandala William Blake's well-known verse: 'For every thing that lives is holy.'[13] But whatever the dramatherapists' religious or spiritual beliefs might be, what they cannot miss is a trust in men and women as creative beings, owning the talent to regenerate themselves:

> The meaning of creativity does not have to be necessarily associated to the great artistic expressions, but to the fact that I, as a single being, can succeed in experimenting with new things, that is to say, succeed in building within my own experience a life dimension in which can be active the same drive that leads or pushes some Leonardo, Michelangelo, Beethoven and Proust, to the creation. [. . .] We must then nerve ourselves and impose on ourselves the assignment of reviving in us the creative dimension, through which we feel alive and free. I use the verb 'revive' not casually. In fact, we can revive only what has been alive; this means that the creative dimension has always existed in our life, since it is a prerogative of humanity, otherwise we would not have the world we have.
>
> (Carotenuto 1991: 552–4)

It can be arduous to recognize Michelangelo in a young man nailed on a wheelchair or Leonardo in a silent figure curled up within herself because of fear of the world, just as it is sometimes even difficult to recognize the creative principle in ourselves, tight as we are in the grip of everyday life 'in which consciences grow mouldy'. But if this trust points the way, allowing us also to nurture hope in failures and disappointments (which, as whoever works in the field of 'helping relationships' well knows, are many and unavoidable), then something will happen sooner or later, and behind grey and dusty masks we will perceive the shine of eyes that are alive and humanly longing for the future.

A similar attitude must go along with respect. If I consider the other as a bearer of the creative principle, I must approach him without judging, and I must try to help him find his own way, neither conditioning him nor overlapping him. This aspect is of particular relevance because drama is an outstandingly powerful tool, with such an evocative strength to rouse violent emotional flows, which can very easily influence people:

> Once someone is engaged in the drama process it is very easy to implant ideas, create auto-suggestions, manipulate memories and

re-create a personality. This is why it is essential that people are properly trained in the use of drama methods and that they also examine their own motives for using drama. It is unacceptable to want to assert power over other people, by making them vulnerable through the drama.

(Jennings 1998: 105)

To observe this precept, we need to have a specific competence in dramatic art; so we go back to the Mandala, to explore the northeast sector, that of *Skills*. Dramatic experience in the first person is important not only because, as I have said before, it puts us in contact with the drama's transformative power, but also because it allows us a direct experimentation with the intimate psycho-physiological mechanisms which are at the roots of that power. For instance, the relationship between gesture, voice and emotional activation; or the dynamic of relaxation/ concentration in the action.

But dramatic knowledge is not enough to guarantee to manage the dramatic process towards an improvement of people's well-being. To 'keep the fire alight', to provide inputs suitable to the different contexts and help addressing the process towards a development, the drama-therapist should be able to understand what happens: to connect people's ways to be present with their personal issues; to identify the positive resources of the subjects; to formulate some hypothesis to interpret the sense that actions, roles, scenes and stories play in the process, both in regard to the individuals, and to the group. To build some good models for grasping reality, we cannot avoid considering what the human sciences (ethology, anthropology, philosophy, sociology, psychology, neuro-sciences) try to tell about this multifaceted biped to whose kind we all belong. There exists also what the poets have sung and dramatists and writers have told: I believe that what Dostoevskij and Thomas Mann can tell us about the secret of the human nature is not less worthy than what Freud or Lévi-Strauss did. Murray Cox, who was a great therapist besides a sensitive researcher of the structures of the healing process, has written:

Shakespeare is an incomparable inspiration in therapeutic work by reason of his deep knowledge of the mind, his poetic language (which uses a wide range of mutually reinforcing symbols and allusions), his playing with metaphors and paradoxes, and his oscillations between concrete and abstract statements. He takes an image, delights in playing with it, and compresses in one short sentence an astonishing wealth of associations.

(Cox and Theilgaard 1994: 328)

Stories, legends, myths, fairytales, with their load of ancient wisdom, distilled through the centuries, enhance our knowledge of human things and open the horizon of symbolic thought, as well as the deepest studies of religions and comparative mythologies (first of all the works of Joseph Campbell).

It is also necessary to recognize that we cannot understand everything. However sophisticated and complex our interpretative tools may be, there will always be a portion of reality that will escape our understanding. It is sometimes rather our excessive certainty in our theories and grids that makes us shortsighted with regard to some aspects of the world that don't fit in our categories. Landy, reflecting upon his own training as a dramatherapist, tells us of his meeting with the certainty/uncertainty polarity as follows:

> 'Certain' therapists were ones who had not only mastered a certain technique or approach, but believed that it was certain to work most of the time. Certainty applied to those psychiatrists, for example, who treated a symptom rather than a person, prescribing medications to quell the hyperactive and stimulate the depressive, those whose treatment was based upon predictable behavioral results. Uncertain therapists were ones who acknowledged the mysteries and the complexities of behavior, thought, feeling, intuition. Uncertain therapists worked with individuals who appear catatonic, ignorant, senile, rigid, self-destructive, totally lost within themselves, and first dared to acknowledge the limits of their techniques and under-standings. Then, engaging their professional skills, they devised strategies, uncertain as to the outcomes. [. . .] I wanted to be both certain and uncertain – a professional certain of his knowledge and of skills, yet open to the uncertainties of the therapeutic process.
>
> (Landy 1996: 73–4)

To recognize and to accept the limits of our own knowledge goes along with accepting our own limits as persons. Here we enter the southeast sector of the Mandala, that of *Vulnerability*. Sometimes, during the dramatic process, images appear that bother us, and we do not succeed in understanding them. The role of sorrowful and subjected mother, despised by husband and children, can be unbearable for me, and I will try to suggest cues to transform it, for instance, into a withstanding mother (as Mother Courage in Brecht's play). But how much of this operation matches with the client's needs, and how much does my impatience come from an unresolved relationship with my own motherly figure? Such a kind of doubt is recurrent in the process, and this is good, because it constantly warns us about the risk of imposing our personal needs on those of the clients, and therefore influencing them, suggesting solutions that can be received but not creatively acknowledged, and therefore become a superficial learning, but not a source of deep change. People perhaps need time to freely express their emotions, with no close necessity to get to a catharsis or to a turning point. A resolution could however come, similar to the one we suggest, and this can make us understand as some aspects of our experience and feelings coincide with those of the client, but it cannot authorize us in any case to step over their needs rather than supporting them. Marina Jenkyns tackles this theme applying the psychoanalytic categories of transference and counter-transference:

> It is crucial that the dramatherapist has extensively explored his or her own inner world through in-depth personal therapy in order to be aware of the possible sources and nature of the of counter-transference reactions.
>
> (Jenkyns 1996: 54)

It is good and helpful to try to know our own dark sides, our unsolved issues and our fears. To know doesn't mean necessarily to remedy: the dramatherapist cannot and must not try to be perfect. He can be and he must be complete instead. To be complete means also to welcome inside our vision of those parts of us whose wounds are not yet healed, and to take care of them. 'Uncle, what does torment you?' This is the question that Parsifal asks the Fisher King, and from which the transformation begins.

To recount our own personal story, telling it to someone who knows how to listen, can be of great use. I always encourage my students, particularly those who operate in the clinical fields (in treatment of mental disorders and addictions, as well as in 'palliative care'), to undergo a thorough individual or group psychotherapy of a 'confessional' type, whatever the theoretical models of reference are (psychoanalysis, analytical psychology, counselling, Gestalt, psychodrama or any other form of psychotherapy: the main point is that the therapist is sensitive and honest). I also find very useful the exercises of autobiographic writing suggested by the pedagogist Duccio Demetrio (1996) and the practice of the Jungian 'active imagination' (see Kast 1988).

The one who can help us better to bear the presence of such different aspects of our soul – that of the confident person, able to help, and that of the vulnerable person who lives with fears and uncertainties, which enable us to share the other's experience – is our artistic part (*Artist* in the southwest sector of the Mandala). It is actually the artistic principle that helps us to bear the ambivalence:

> The creative choice involves my maintaining the tension among the contraries. Those contraries, brought back to the key principles, are good and evil, God and the devil. There were religions for which the evil and the good represented two faces of the same divinity. [. . .] The creative man, in other terms, accepts living the conflict.
>
> (Carotenuto 1991: 468)

I could add, returning to the cultural horizon of Dramatherapy, that according to Landy, one of the primary therapeutic aims of the dramatic process is helping people to bear role ambivalence in everyday life.[14]

Artists are persons on the border; for them the tension among the contraries is the source of creative energy, the synthesis or the transcendence of them the goal of the creative process. From the synthesis springs the newness: the glance of the artist goes through the chaos and finds some forms in it. The internal creative artist must be fed. It is a good habit for the dramatherapist to practise at least another artistic discipline besides the theatre (and not necessarily connected with it), as well as to enjoy all the arts. He should also take time to gaze at the sea or the clouds, the bugs or the rocks; to play with a cat or with a child; to grant himself moments of idleness and of what Gaston Bachelard called *poetic rêverie* (1960).

The last sector of the Mandala is that of the *Guide*. This aspect is particularly complex. On the one hand it concerns the attitude to observe our own actions from an 'external' point of view that the dramatherapist must constantly maintain: a regular supervision of the daily work helps in developing this attitude, as well as mastering and sharpening our own tools.[15] On the other hand, it suggests that we start listening to our deep images and deciphering their messages, trusting an internal wisdom that is a gift given to every creature, and which waits only to be unearthed. Practices of psycho-physical concentration (such as Yoga, T'ai Chi Ch'uan or Vipassana meditation) can help us to maintain an 'internal breath' and a serenity of mind essential to face situations of suffering and desolation so hard to bear.

Mandala exercise

I would like to conclude this chapter with a simple imaginative exercise which I would suggest that the readers try for themselves.[16] First of all, we have to draw the Mandala. We need a sheet of paper, a pencil, a rubber, a felt pen, a compass, a ruler and a setsquare. We can proceed by tracing the external circle, marking the centre and the vertical diameter of it, then the external square and the horizontal diameter, and therefore the smaller circle (it can be done far more quickly with the computer, but I believe that the concentration strength for the realization of the pattern is a good introduction to the relaxation required by the middle part of the exercise). You can then trace the figure of the Mandala with the pen and cancel the extra lines of pencil.

Let's now set our attention on the smallest circle in the centre: it is what concerns the values that sustain our world vision. Let's try to synthesize this vision into a single sentence. We can take as long as we need. When we have found a sentence that satisfies us, let's write it in the centre of the circle. At this point, we must take into account the four sectors: our knowledge and our abilities; our vulnerability; our artistic part; our internal guide. We can colour them with watercolours. This technique allows us to play on the nuances. (I suggest, however, to those who are not familiar with watercolour to test it first on another sheet.) We can now close our eyes and try to empty our minds, keeping our concentration on the breath. We can try to imagine the air entering from the right nostril, filling our whole body and going out from the left nostril; then it enters again from the left nostril, fills and goes out from the right one: the cycle can be repeated 14 times (seven for each nostril). If we feel relaxed enough, we can try, always with our eyes closed, to visualize the Mandala and to imagine, for every sector, a character that represents it. These can be fictional characters, from a novel or play, from a fairytale, film or even a comic strip. They can be famous people or someone we know personally; or can simply be made up right now. We can give some features to these characters, trying to visualize their characteristics. Now, let's imagine that these characters speak to us and that each one of them utters a sentence addressed to us at this moment. Then we open our eyes, take the pen and we begin to count aloud from 100 to zero. During this countdown, we can write the sentences that we have listed in the four sectors of the Mandala in the order we prefer. The counting can be repeated twice if the time is not enough (but I suggest not more). We now observe the Mandala again, reading the sentences we have written. Perhaps we will only find confirmations of things that we already know, but we may discover some elements that may catch us, and upon which it is worthwhile reflecting.

Part III

Dramatherapy and its applications

Dramatherapy is a therapy of optimism; it is a therapy of now and the future; it is able to assist people to move on, rather than perpetually delve into an unhelpful past.

(Sue Jennings 1998)

Chapter 5

Mental health

> Cowper[1] came to me and said, 'Oh! That I were insane, always . . . Oh!
> that in the bosom of God I was hid. You retain health, and yet are mad
> as any of us all – over us all – mad as a refuge from unbelief . . .
> (William Blake, Marginalium to Spurzheim,
> *Observations on Insanity*, 1817)

Mad people and us

It took almost three centuries from when we had begun to confine mad
people (in leper hospitals, jails, general hospitals or special structures)
to devise a science to deal with this specific problem. Therefore, most of
our knowledge of the world of those people we called from time to time
mad, crazy, fool, mentally ill or psychotic stems from observations 'in
captivity', within the frame of an asymmetrical relationship between a
free person and one who is not.[2]

The asymmetry of a relationship (also defined in terms of power and
influence) is likely to produce complementary rigid roles; one (the 'down'
role) is established in regard to the other (the 'up' role), and is modified
by redefinitions of the situation made by the 'up' role. The feedback of
these modifications tends to influence the 'up' role, provoking a further
change, but the possibility that this may happen is connected with the
control that the 'up' role sets upon the 'down' role. A model of this
dynamic is the father–child relationship: accepting the transformations of
the other in terms of autonomy, increasingly relinquishing control,
modifies the fatherly role. The roles gain symmetry, until there is
recognition of a new relationship between adults. A stiffening of the role,
in terms of 'wanting not to release the control', produces the withdrawal
of the authorization and stops the possibility of growth, or reduces it to
an expedient for survival.

In the context of an institution whose principle purpose is control (a purpose that is a basic condition with which the psychiatrist is not able to disagree, even if as a doctor his professional objective is healing), the roles must remain rigid or else the institution itself will collapse. Over a long period (almost more than three centuries) in which the pair of psychiatrist/asylum has been indissoluble, 'mad' has become 'ill'. As Michel Foucault stated, before the Age of the Enlightenment reason conversed with madness.[3] The mad person's role in theatre, according to Landy's 'taxonomy of roles', 'reveals the dark, shadowy sides of human nature and challenges the conventional notion of sanity'. 'Ill people', on the other hand, are those who need to be taken care of, and that therefore cannot fundamentally take care of themselves or of the others. Those who have met people who lived for a long time in asylums know the efforts made to stick to such a role, which have been able to guarantee them surviving there. Erving Goffman, in *Asylums* (1961), where he continues his investigation into social performance that he started with *The Presentation of Self in Everyday Life* (1959), describes the moral career of the mentally ill, from the circumstances marking the beginning of it (which are often set as a sort of dramatic performance), to the adaptation to the 'ward system', reconstructing a new identity, so intensely mirrored and strengthened by the surrounding structure to become definitive.[4]

Mentally ill Persona

I will never forget my first meetings with Matteo, 40 years an inmate of the 'Pietro Pisani' asylum in Palermo. When I met him, he was a tall and large man, about 70 years old but still at the height of his strength, who nonetheless looked wrinkled, retreated into himself. He walked hanging his head, shuffling his feet, and he seemed so much smaller than he was. When a group of in-patients passed together along the long avenue of the hospital, one would have difficulty in distinguishing them. It looked as if even their bodies were fitted only for that, ineluctable Persona of the 'mentally ill', walking with their heads hanging and shuffling their feet. A body deserted by a shattered Self can be easily invaded by a very powerful Persona. Matteo's body embodied the mentally ill Persona to the point that his own skin was as grey as the suits of raw cloth that he wore. His slow, heavy movements, tending to unbalance, amplified the side effects of the medicines he had taken for so many years. He talked a lot, minutely telling all the details of his day: the awakening, what he had eaten at breakfast, the medicines he had taken, how he had got dressed and whom he had met or seen. He had been a cobbler in his youth, in a small Sicilian village and, it seems, a happy and sociable man. After a shameful incident (his bride ran away with a man belonging to a mafia family), he started to do strange things. He didn't sleep at night, he went around dirty and torn, he sang obscene songs in the street. Then he had been arrested (it was in the early 1950s) and therefore interned. During the first years he had often succeeded in escaping from the insane asylum, making long trips, but he always came back. Yet he seemed a man without a story.

Rita, a nurse, ran an 'occupational therapy workshop' – the only place where the in-patients could meet outside the wards. When they came in the morning, Rita made them have a wash and supplied them with normal clothes. On the wall of the long and narrow hall where people did hand crafts or simply stayed together for part of the day, before going back to their wards, Rita had nailed an old map of Italy, a little worn-out one, but still with bright colours. Matteo used to stare at it for a long time. Then he started to list the regions and their chief towns, passing on to Europe and the world. He ended by asking me to ask him questions on the capitals of some almost unknown countries, which he always answered correctly. Warmed by this sketch of communication, Matteo started again to speak. This time streams of things came out of his world in a chaotic and disconnected way. He mixed 'memory and desire', as Eliot says. He mingled life episodes and imaginings. He sang mangled songs, putting personal facts into them. He overlapped people in the hospital with people from his own past. Talking, he left behind that wrinkled and taut aspect and even began to have a light colour to his cheeks. He was more human, but more incomprehensible. Behind the Persona (the submissive and accommodating ill person, alomost obsessively respectful of the rules), a rich and complex world emerged, but crumbled and upset, with its own grammar, impossible to decipher.

The passage from considering the Persona to meeting the experience of mentally ill people leads on the one hand to the break-up of the determinations that sustains control (the definition in comparison to the norm, for instance) and on the other hand it gives room to the possibility for a searching of sense in the apparently foolish manifestations of madness; for a new hermeneutics that not only acknowledges the symptoms as signs of a lack, but also as elements of constructs contrived to meet the world. Constructs that are ruinous, in the sense that they conduct to an isolation of the person as they are not comprehensible according to the common sense, but that had became, as Arieti writes, 'his way to enter in relationship with the others and to interpret the world' (1959–66: 584).

The great attempt on the part of psychiatry of the last century, from the 1960s onwards,[5] to reconsider mentally ill people as persons and, accordingly, try to make sense of their experience, grew along with the political and cultural striving to give them back their human dignity. This attempt also passed through the non-medical approaches to psychiatry derived from phenomenology, psychoanalysis and communication theories, proposing psycho-social explanations of the aetiology of the psychosis, rather than biological. This trend led to the closing of the insane asylums and to the refocusing of psychiatric work on 'mental health' rather on 'illness'.[6] In Italy, the so-called Basaglia Law, from the name of the psychiatrist who, more than any other, fought against the inhuman treatment meted out to mentally ill people, dates back to 1978.

Body and psychosis

The difficulty of such a meeting is the incommensurability between our way of adaptation to the world (which we define normal, in the sense of recognition and acceptance of the norms, at least in the behavioural appearance) and that of the person living the psychotic condition. Its importance is in the respect for the person through the whole acceptance of their condition, even if it is not possible to understand it completely (bearing therefore the presence of an area of 'secret' (see Zapparoli 1987). This involves the principle that healing is not reduced to the abolition of symptoms and the adjustment to a prearranged model (the idea of 'normality' recognized by the institution), as in the pharmacotherapy/ rehabilitation scheme, but that it is a process aimed at facilitating the reorganization of the person, beginning from their own resources and from their way of being in that condition, and therefore to a reduction of their suffering coming from the act of accepting the world, rather than withdrawing from it, as in illness.

Psychotic condition is expressed, in fact, through the body. The body of a psychotic person conveys to us a sense of uneasiness, not because it is a sick body but because it speaks with an extreme language, alluding to the extreme degrees of identity. Sometimes the body of the psychotic person is far away. It is like an object without life and without importance, from which something that once could say 'I am this' has withdrawn for a long time. Galimberti has written:

> When the body is not lived anymore as my *subjectivity*, but, outdis-
> tanced from me, is *objectified* and reduced to the dimension of an
> anatomical body, to which the internal self imputes what is for him

the tragic condition to be seen and heard, then the refusal of the body becomes symbol of the greatest refusal, investing society, solidarity with the others, appointment in the world. [. . .] The withdrawal from the body is therefore withdrawal from the world.

(Galimberti 1983: 180)

The objectification of the body in search of a possible form of atharaxy (imperturbability) or apathy (absence of emotions), of an end to the pain through annulment of the senses, which has been described as the 'petrifying' of the psychotic condition, is the reaction to a mimetic engulfment one is not allowed to get rid of, in which the body is felt as being nude and vulnerable, defenceless from the wounds of the world, crossed by intolerable emotional discharges. The alternative is its destruction: self-injury, anorexia and suicide go in this direction.

In the tension between wounded body and petrified body, the possibility to articulate one's own mimetic relationships with others is blocked. The ability to govern the boundaries between oneself and the world are lost and the distinctions between inside and outside, reality and fancy, words and things, become confused and blurred.

Threshold work

Dramatic work is, to a greater extent, an establishment of boundaries. The intention is not to maintain them in a defensive sense but to cross them at will, achieving new awareness in crossing them. The dramatic agreement is based upon a particular meta-communicative clarity, which can be underlined by a specific connotation of the space as a dramatic space, with a separation between 'stage' – the area of 'as if' – and 'audience' – the area of 'here and now' – and it must be maintained and strengthened throughout the whole process. The protection from invasion by the other is guaranteed, as the meaningful interactions between people are contained in a frame ('this is a play' or 'this is drama'), recognizable both through its definition by statements and spatial denotations, and through the action. The therapist must be the 'guarantor of the thresholds', as it is only when the equilibrium is preserved that the process can be set out. He needs, therefore, to draw on his own aesthetical sense and theatrical competence to perceive the dissonances in crossing borders, as well as his own empathy to understand the sense of them in relation to the suffering expressed by the psychotic person, and his own creativity to devise and suggest ways to recover dissonance in a healing sense.

David Read Johnson identifies the relationship of person/role within improvisation as a place in which threshold dissonance becomes visible to the dramatic eye. He sets out a model of dramatic interaction that includes four levels:

A) *Impersonal*: the relationship between two enacted roles (e.g. between the salesman and the customer);
B) *Intrapersonal*: the relationship between each person and his own role (e.g. between Bob and the salesman, and Jane and the customer);
C) *Extrapersonal*: the relationship between each person and the other's person role (e.g. between Bob and the customer and Jane and the salesman);
D) *Interpersonal*: the relationship between the two individuals (e.g. between Bob and Jane).

(in Schattner and Courtney 1981: 53)

Each of these interaction levels is a meaningful threshold area, with its own specific problems. Johnson suggests that there is a minimum level of cognitive and emotional clarity for the drama to be possible. If there is a consistent difficulty with the boundaries in the impersonal or in the interpersonal area, for example, if the subject mistakes himself for the other or the role of the other (Bob acts as if he were Jane, or as if he were the client), it means that the dimension of the 'as if' is totally inaccessible. 'Confusions of this kind', writes Johnson, 'should not be allowed to continue, and may indicate that the patient is currently too disorganized to benefit from role playing' (ibid.: 55). Confusion in the other threshold areas is, on one hand, the signal of a difficulty on the axis of distance (tending to overdistancing or underdistancing), reflecting a particular way of meeting the world; on the other hand it expresses a possible interpretation/performance in a specifically theatrical sense, which is able to be changed. The intervention can assume the form of a cognitive tuning that helps to correct the balance of the person/role relationship through an examination of difficulties and possible corrective suggestions. It may also be necessary to insist on threshold demarcations, together with inter- ventions about the space or with specific dramatic actions (intensification or lightening of the emotional load of the role). These interventions are an immediate redefinition of the situation that can also happen within the dramatic sequence, having the function of instant feedback. They are necessary when the difficulty in distancing blocks the scene, provoking a performance short circuit. For instance, when the subject can't play a role because the fear of being submerged by it sets up a state of anxiety, it may be right to carry on with the scene by loosening the tension – perhaps introducing a comic element – thus offering the person the possibility of keeping the drama flowing and to talk about it later. Alternatively, when the subject lacks the ability to concentrate and to focus on the particular role he is playing, and he is confined to 'playing himself' more or less faithfully, he can be helped to work on the correct balance with some technical tool such as the development of the character in time or space, the *a parte* or the soliloquy.[7]

These interventions are on the polarity of the feedback:[8] the modification of an event or a sequence of actions within the progress of them, caused by the influence of information that is present. In our case, it means managing the thresholds in the concreteness of the single case. This provides an immediate awareness, generating an enhancement of the performance ability; for example, the management in a coherent way of a difficult role (because it is emotionally weighted or because it bears uncomfortable analogies with our difficulties in everyday life). The feedback intervention can lead to an insight, an instant visualization of the problematic knot, but it may not ensure a rebalancing of the person that can go beyond the sphere of pertinence of the single occurrence toward a general restructuring of the threshold constructs. In other words, I may be able to play a role in which an emotion (for instance, fear) can be controlled, but I might not be able to control the fear itself. The repetition of feedback interventions, calibrated on specific individual problems, is an educational feature of Dramatherapy, similar to Moreno's role training (see Moreno 1946: 201).[9] This approach is useful in creating the conditions for the transformation process to trigger: for instance, to allow the subject progressively to free himself from the 'ill' role and begin to think of himself as someone worthy of being trusted, able to communicate and to undertake relationship.

Bearing confusion

It is also important to bear elements of disorientation or confusion, which can be functional for a self-presentation reflecting the actual condition of the person: their state of mind, their relational world and their self-image. N is a 15-year-old girl, who has been attending the centre for a year with a diagnosis of borderline personality disorders. She has suffered from epilepsy since early childhood, which has not jeopardized her cognitive faculties but has led to the construction of a negative self-image of an ugly, stupid and incapable person with an asexual body. This is compensated somehow with obsessive rituals (which in adolescence turned into a maniacal passion for jigsaw puzzles and the construction of houses of cards). We are at the first meeting after the summer break. During the conversation before the drama session, N proposes to talk about what we did in the summer. I accept the proposal, even though we had already talked about this topic during the reception process before the workshops started. I suggest that we use drama rather than words to do it. When her turn arrives, N seems at first incapable of remembering any episode of her summer worthy to be staged. P, another girl in the group who is always very careful about personal life details, reminds her that her birthday was in August. So N tells us that she went to a pizzeria with her relatives. She then sets the scene by putting all the chairs side by side, like a school rather than a restaurant. In giving the roles, N is rather generic. It is neither clear whether the characters are real or invented (she speaks of a 24-year-old nephew), nor is it clear what her relationship with them is, nor the affective relevance she ascribes to them. The moment to order the meal arrives and N rises from the guest of honour seat and takes the orders. Then she stands up to fetch the pizzas and even to cook them herself. From a strictly theatrical point of view this is a rough error that should be corrected. (Furthermore, in going to the kitchen, N crosses the imaginary table that she herself had created.) It also needs correction because it is confirmation of a substantial dispersion of N's identity, which is one of the signs of her pathology. The scene could be stopped, to focus the confusion point, and repeated with the correction made. But could it not be that this confusion is for her somehow functional in keeping her own person? In this case, a denial of it could be a disconfirmation of the person, like those N is used to receiving from her family and the social environment. The escape from the guest of honour seat is perhaps a demonstration of an incapability to bear emotions and affection because of the fear of emotional overwhelming; a defensive structure that N carries on and that denies for her the possibilities of relationships, connected with a fundamental disesteem for herself: I am unworthy to be celebrated. On the other hand, it is also directed toward a different possibility of role (the role of the person useful to others, even if only practically, without affective involvement) that N had already mentioned in a previous performance, when she played the role of a social worker for elderly people, commenting that this is a job she would be eager to do.

These subroles, expressing fantasies or potentialities, have right of citizenship. We have to give room to them, even if they are used as escapes from roles that in normality would be more suitable (the role of the teenager celebrating her birthday among loving friends) but that at present, at least in real life, are not feasible. In drama perhaps they are.

After the pizzas and the drinks have been taken to the table, I suggest to N: 'Now you could sit and eat your pizza.' The scene that follows is an amusing game of mutual tasting of bits of pizza. N has returned to the place of honour, this time with a more relaxed bodily attitude, and takes part in the party. The transformation to waitress, which at first had baffled us a little because of the too sudden change, has conveyed a more complex image of N to the group, in which the difficulty to be inside an affective network is expressed along with a desire of being accepted by the others. The roles of the other participants become more generic, less tied to real characters of the event (supposing that the first ones were real and not just embodiments of meaningless relationships). It is easier to put into them parts of ourselves that can nurture N in the difficult task of healing the wounds of lack of love. In the second part of the day N attends the pottery group and for the first time in almost a year she neither asks 'What shall I do?' nor violently bangs her piece of clay on the table making everybody jump. Surprisingly, she creates a tiny funny face: her first human figure.

Heaven and hell

The dramatic process develops therefore in a delicate balance between corrective interventions and spaces in which the subjects can express 'ill' parts of themselves with no fear of being judged, authorized by a 'good enough' group, which can accept and bear the defects and lacks of its members. 'Mutual forgiveness of each vice: these are the gates of Paradise' wrote Blake.

The dramatic reality built up in the group, as unusual and eccentric as it may be, is nevertheless communicable, and therefore shareable. Imagination, and therefore the creative part of the person, overcomes the condition of *adualism*, becoming a relational and socially mediated dimension. Through it, the existential nuclei of the person, even if linked to extreme forms of adaptation, find a metaphoric possibility of being revealed, in the shape of images that become common heritage, breaking the chains of isolation and showing themselves as places of encounter.

I would like to end this section with a last short story. We are at the fifteenth meeting of a one-year Dramatherapy cycle with the outpatients of an adult psychiatric day hospital. The group has been fluctuating, even though a nucleus of four or five people have been attending all the sessions. Among them there is S, a 24-year-old man of fair though untidy appearance, with a stiff and self-folded bodily attitude. S has spent his childhood and adolescence within the boundaries of an orphanage, where he had begun a bright sporting career as a boxer that was slashed – a few years after his discharging from the institute – by alcohol and a series of delirious episodes over the last years. He lives alone upon a small disability pension, without any social relationships. That morning during the warm-up, I noticed in him an unusual intolerance of collaborating with the others and a certain general resistance to share. When we were seated in a circle, I asked him to think of an image that could express his internal state at this moment. 'I feel as a bomb, rather, an atomic bomb; I feel I could explode and destroy the whole world.' We set up the scene. S stands on a high spot on stage, ready to fall upon the world. The other group members build the world that will be destroyed. Everyone takes up a role and the social interactions begin. On the stage S can't make up his mind to act. I ask him if he would like to stop the scene. 'No, no,' he answers, 'I was just looking. Now I am going to explode.' And indeed he explodes, but it is such a tiny bang that the world is not destroyed. The others complain. They don't feel motivated to the apocalypse if the explosion is not impressive enough. S explodes again, and this time it is an overwhelming event. All the people are physically touched and they die, each one in his own way. At this point, we cannot but give a glance to the afterlife. We all move onto the stage, with S as a judge who, after a brief interview, sends the characters to hell or to heaven (as is easy to imagine, purgatory is not taken into consideration). When the judgement comes to an end, the situation seems to become sluggish. The world has ended, we are all dead and we are not better or worse than before. S, who had been very excited during the scene, now seems rather exhausted.

The group feels a moment of perplexity, soon interrupted by C, another patient, proposing, 'Why don't we play a football match between angels and devils?' He offers to make a running commentary on the event, the teams are formed and the match can begin. It goes on for almost a quarter of an hour with both patients and staff busy chasing and striking an imaginary ball with all the enthusiasm and involvement of a group of boys that have finally found a meadow in which to play football with friends. There is no referee because S, when asked by a companion, answers that he prefers to play and is co-opted as a midfield player by the team of devils. I don't remember the score of the game, nor who won. I can only testify that at the end of the scene, after a short de-roling, the group warmly thanked S and everybody greeted each other with great friendliness. Along the road back to the day hospital, the group walked quietly, chatting of religion and of sport, with S and C walking arm in arm like old friends.

Chapter 6

Addictions

And if unluckily it should happen, in any way, anything unpleasant, well, there is always the *soma* that allows you a vacation away from the real facts. And there is always the *soma* to calm your anger, to reconcile you with your enemies, to make you patient and tolerant. In the past these things could not happen but with great efforts and after years of painful moral training. Now two or three tablets of half a gram, and everything is all right.

(Aldous Huxley, *The Brave New World*, 1932)

The weight of the world

'When the rich were taking drugs, it was picturesque. When the poor take drugs, it is a national scourge.' This is the caption of a caustic cartoon by the French humorist Reiser that compares the image of an elegant gentleman smoking a pipe of opium in quiet solitude in a room with exotic furniture with the image of many young people, ugly and dirty, with a rather depressed look, crowded in a bleak hall. The cartoon dates back to the beginning of the 1970s and, reconsidered now, it looks ominously prophetic. At that time the use of 'hard drugs', those which cause addiction,[1] was the prerogative of small elites who somehow still maintained a certain romantic conception of drug use, in which the substance is experienced as a door to a world of ecstasy and imagination, like opium for De Quincey and hashish for Baudelaire. But an era of the mass spreading of drugs was impending: heroin from the East and cocaine from South America were starting to invade the Western world, tied up with criminal affairs and interwoven with the harsh politics of dominion and terror.[2] The youth countercultures that had tried an 'assault to the sky', bringing into question those values of progress, consumption and indiscriminate growth which were more and more revealing themselves to be arid and deeply inhuman, were crumbling, leaving a frightened and uneasy generation, with an identity so frail that it often ruinously surrendered to the flatteries of the 'artificial paradises'.[3]

Along with the growth of availability, the areas of consumption extended beyond the disappointed rebels and decadent aesthetes to touch the suburbs, the spots of discomfort and social alienation that the opulent society attempted in vain to hide or forget. On the threshold of the 1980s, the phenomenon of drug addiction was already a cause for social alarm, producing thousands of corpses every year and triggering a heavy increase in juvenile delinquency, while the international drug trafficking was kept firmly in the hands of powerful, many-branched criminal organizations.[4]

The actions of social and sanitary institutions, as well as those of the repressive apparatuses, do not seem to have stemmed the phenomenon; rather it has spread, increased in later years by the diffusion of so-called 'new drugs', connected with ritual mass behaviours of young people; drugs that are seemingly harmless, but whose effects are proving to be just as destructive.

It has been argued that if the use of heroin and similar drugs was not so tightly caught up in a vicious circle of micro-crime (the consumer who steals, becomes a prostitute, or a drug pusher to get his daily fix), making the phenomenon evident to everybody, we probably would not pay so much attention to it. After all the threshold of tolerance for alcoholism, which has an even older history, has been rising, despite the fact that its effects on the health of the people involved are just as ruinous. There is no doubt that after the failure of repression politics (prison for drug addicts) and of internment politics (coercive therapeutic communities), we have reached a state of fatalistic resignation that in these last years has taken the name of 'damage reduction'. Considering the difficulty of recovering the addicts and the total impossibility of stopping the expansion of dependence habits, we just try to limit the damage both to the consumer and to the community. The main way to put this strategy into practice is to substitute the addictive substance (usually heroin) with another, supplied under medical control. It avoids the risk that greater physical damage (from illnesses transmitted by needles, or the lethal effects of substances used to adulterate the drug) can afflict the addicts. Besides, it allows them to leave the spiral of trafficking and the constant need for money and avoids their ending up in the nets of the criminal underworld.

But the whole process is like trying to hold water in a basket: the problem escapes from everywhere, producing new rivulets which are equally upsetting. We have discovered, for instance, that almost half of the addicts in care in the public services show consistent symptoms of personality disorders (psychotic and borderline). It almost seems that the substance has been chosen as an unaware autotherapy, to bear an inner deflagration, otherwise unbearable, which comes to the surface unchanged, if not worsened, when this coverage fades away.

Actually, the cycle of the heroin can overwhelm the whole person. The first effect of a heroin puncture is a feeling of engulfment – the *flash*[5] and the *planet*[6] – in which the self expands to the point of dissolving, leaving behind all suffering and pain. Even desire is gone. The ecstatic condition is enough in itself, it doesn't need anything, not even the body, and it doesn't desire anything. But the desire returns powerfully when the biochemical effect of the substance weakens, in the *descent* phase.[7] The body is perceived again as a burden of grief to drag around, victim of all the wounds of the world, and the whole individual identity is subdued by the need, creating a rigid Persona, one dimensional and all involving, permeating all the expressions of individual life. 'Junk is not a kick, it is a way of living' was the verdict of William Burroughs, the 'drug addict *par excellence*' (quoted in Wilshire 1998: xv).

This flattening of identity within a unique process that becomes recursive, self-referring and self-reproducing annuls the possibilities of a creative relationship with the world. When the world returns, it is threatening and unfriendly. This perception is promptly mirrored by the social context: the label of ex-addict dies hard and it is often the only element upon which one can reconstruct a social status.

Out of the circle, the soul is naked and brittle as crystal. It can shatter at every bump and it is not elastic enough to contrive new forms of adaptation. But the lack of that form of protection, caused by the annulment of consciousness and body awareness, reveals above all another much deeper lack, echoed in the pain of the descent from the drug, and of which one becomes tragically aware, even unable to name it.

What we miss

Trying to give a name to this lack means trying to understand the reasons that push people to addiction. It allows us to reflect on a crucial point: does a specific pathology of drug addiction exist? That is to say, can we identify a particular structuring of the person that invariably leads to the objected condition, or is drug addiction only a variation on a larger theme, embracing a range of potential existences that reach all of us?

Research has pointed out affective disorders of the first childhood, in the area of what Bowlby (1973) calls 'anxious attachment'. A Buddhist master once told me of a meditation experience with addict inmates in a New Zealand prison. Within a meditation path, he proposed an exercise in which the subject is asked internally to turn toward himself with the fond attitude of a mother toward her own children. But the search of an inner maternal world collided with the bleakness of the experience. 'If I should meet my mother now, at least I would beat her up' – such were the inmates' comments about their own difficulty in carrying out the exercise. Not to be nurtured, or swinging between a nurturing missed or only mimed and 'an intrusive nurturing, possessive and loaded with frustration, turning a deep interpersonal relationship into an instrumental connection' (Gerra and Frati 2000), jeopardizes the possibility of transitionality, and therefore of a separation doing not too much damage. If the transitional space is not available, mimetic differentiation is incomplete and the ability to master the emotional flows is blocked.

But perhaps lack of love is at the root of all the psychic troubles and sufferings of our age. The affective model enlightens some aspects of the problem, but it does not explain the specificity of the evolution of uneasiness into drug addiction. Imbalances of this kind can evolve into delinquent behaviours, neurosis and psychosis, normal unhappiness, and also addictions. If we extend the area of our reflection we have to consider the fact that in our society addictions are so many: besides drugs and alcohol, and other drugs like coffee and tobacco, considered less harmful or tolerated because of strong economic interests involving governments and the powerful multinational societies, we speak of gambling addicts, sex addicts and work addicts. People can be also addicted to medicines of any type, shopping, television and, more recently, video games and the internet. Perhaps, the opulent society of which Marcuse spoke is a society of addicts. Wilshire speaks of 'ecstasy deprivation' as the supreme sin of a civilization that has turned its back on the holiness of the nature:

> Today in late twentieth century North Atlantic culture we are masters of engineering, the beneficiaries of manifold technologies for achieving things desired, self-advertising paragons of management and control. Many problems yield before the technology: eliminating plaque on the teeth, inoculating against polio, putting persons on the moon, etc. But many people feel dissatisfied and needy. Their lives are flat. They experience ecstasy deprivation and very often addiction.
> (Wilshire 1998: 4)

Ecstatic experience, according to Wilshire, is what both brings us out of ourselves and reconnects us with the deep sources of our being in the world, tied to the boundless inheritance of our kind, of which the civilization that began from the Neolithic age to build walls and tools is only a small part. Without this experience, which partially remains only in art and religion, we lose the sense of our connection with a larger meaning that enfolds all creatures and the whole universe, so we cling to the possession of objects (including other people) to exorcize our finitude and separateness. The lack of ecstasy remains as an unsatisfied need: Aldous Huxley had discussed the 'need, deeply rooted in man, of self-transcendence' and man's 'natural reluctance to undertake the arduous ascent and his search for some false liberation' (1952: 307). According to Huxley, the search for upward transcendence, the spiritual way, is difficult and fatiguing. We therefore invented some shortcuts, which lead us to a rejection of the self, dragging it toward the bottom: 'what seems a god, is actually a demon, what seems a liberation is actually an enslavement. Self-transcendence is invariably descending toward a state less that human' (ibid.: 309). Among these paths of downward self-transcendence, Huxley identifies 'mass elation'[8] and 'elementary sexuality,'[9] besides, of course, the intoxication of alcohol and drugs.

Rebirth strategies

In traditional cultures, ritual provides the movement of expansion and reconnection. In the rites of passage from childhood to adulthood, the subject is disrobed of his child identity and put in connection with the symbolic roots of the community: the ancestors, the guides and the myths. Following this experience he returns, transformed, into the society where he finds his new adult status. In the modern world, the thresholds are more hazy and uncertain. We have invented a potentially endless adolescence, extending far beyond the puberty phase. It has become more a way of being than an age of life. In it, the misadventures of the quest for identity – from levelling out to self-deception, from dismay to disintegration – find an oddly enlarged stage. They are consumed in individual or collective weary plays, not always leading to happy endings. According to the Jungian psychoanalyst Luigi Zoja, drug addiction can be seen as a sort of degenerated initiation, in which the process of transformation connected with the death/rebirth cycle is deformed into *death of rebirth*. But at the roots of what Zoja calls toxic initiation, the primary need remains for a ritual that can enact a new identity, especially when the mimetic structures founding the person are both impelling and frail (unstable equilibriums that hide affective deprivation). The fact that the soul's lacks (the ecstasy deprivation, the need for self-transcendence, the need for ritual) lead to more violent lacks – to devastation and the abyss – is the drug's great deception. We must however reflect on the deep sense of this motivation, which is anyway a tension toward a more complete wholeness of life. Zoja writes:

> If indeed at the hearth of the initiation to drug there is a need to transcend oneself and a nostalgia of the sacred, then also the liberation from it can be reached with a correspondent leap, transcending the preceding situation. Here's the root of the failure of so many therapies primarily founded upon the detoxification: we cannot just eliminate something, we need to project the person toward a completely new dimension.
>
> (Zoja 1985: 19)

How can drama help to make this necessary leap; not to find again a former self that was lost in darkness, but to create a new one? How can drama provide both a support for emotional difficulties and a ritual in which one can leave behind one's own provisional identity in order to expand it and recover it at a new level of integration? As in the field of mental disorders, even here, given the complexity of the problem, any one approach is not enough, and healing can come only from an integration of methods, tools and theories encompassing the problematic areas as much as possible.[10]

My hypothesis is that Dramatherapy can provide a specific contribution to the healing process, by virtue of its ritual nature and its attention to imaginative processes.

Falling

The 'trust games' are a set of exercises largely used in drama training and in educational and therapeutic applications of theatre.[11] They are exercises of great emotional suggestion in which one or more participants, bandaged or with closed eyes, rely on others' care. One of the best known is the 'pendulum game' (otherwise known as 'Joe Egg' or 'trust circle'). In it the participants are divided into small groups (from five to seven people) forming a compact circle. In turn, each of the participants can go to the centre of the circle, close his eyes, oscillate, and finally let himself fall into the others' arms, which will sustain him and gently bring him back to the central position, from which he will be able to fall again.

The loss of the balance here is a real loss, with no pretence elements, and sets off elementary emotional reactions connected with the most archaic of the emotions: fear. Among all the primary emotions, fear is the one that more directly talks with the native voice of the human condition. It is tightly tied to the body and associated with the survival of the kind. The emotion of fear is perceived at an unaware level and can set in motion prodigious energies, which allowed our ancestors to face the danger or promptly to escape it. But it can also totally destroy the will and the abilities of reaction. Challenging fear is the gesture that, in rites of passage, allows meeting the ritual death. In many traditional ceremonies, the participants are dreadfully frightened before undertaking the transformation journey. Similarly, in heroin initiation, bearing the hole and the blood is a proof of courage requested from whoever wants to cross the threshold and go toward the ecstatic experience, which is also a little death. It annuls the world and the pain (anxiety, boredom and fear itself), to drag people into a dimension without borders and categories.

In the game, the initial fear of falling down is soon counterbalanced with a pleasant feeling of being accepted and sustained. The whole community cares for the falling person, avoiding hurting them, cradling and cuddling them and somehow nurturing them. In a workshop with young adults in the detoxification phase, this game was intentionally selected as a test for admittance to the group. 'You have to pass the test' people said to the new group member, echoing a well-known language, and the challenge was always accepted.

The fear/pleasure dynamics are present however in the whole dramatic process. If the fear to fall, which is the core of the game described above, is joined with a neuro-sensorial activation (and the game is perceived as a metaphor of the experience), it is the dramatic experience itself that becomes fear in the moment of performance. In the dramatic action, I have to expose myself, with my body and its mimetic nerves, being sometimes unhealed wounds, and with my expressive abilities, worn out during my permanence in the toxic universe. What can a person expose whose identity, body, conscience and affections have been for long years confined within a wretched Persona from which he is painstakingly trying to get out? In a 'talk show' improvisation, almost all the group members introduced themselves as characters that had just returned from many years of living in foreign countries, and they told their needs and projects. Being somebody else sets people free from the fear and from the suffering to be ourselves, opening the possibility of the being-together game. Roger Grainger has written:

> The effect of this institutionalised masking of the personal identity is to lessen the pressure upon individuals to cling to their own private

disguises, and particularly the defensiveness which prevents them from expressing emotion themselves and causes them to flee from the potentially devastating force of other people's feelings. Nothing which happens within the drama is as dangerous as it would be outside the charmed circle, precisely because it isn't really 'I' to whom it is happening: and yet it is sufficiently 'I' to make me laugh at what is going on between these people; and sometimes cry a little too.

(in Jennings 1992: 175)

The pleasure to create, to build worlds, for the simple fact that it is a game whose heart is liberty, is a pleasure that leaves neither a bitter taste in people's mouths, nor the loneliness of the day after, but the feeling of a corporate experience. A group member comments at the end of the Dramatherapy cycle: 'I don't know if it is the same for the others: I have ascertained that I feel very good here. I feel like. . .home. . .like. . .in a family. . .I don't know how to explain it. . .I have grown fond of this group as much as the members of my family.'

The voices of the spirits

A: (*To himself, on the edge of the moulding*) I can't bear this life any more. It is disgusting. Life is a shit.

B (*Entering on stage with an unmistakable pregnant tummy*): Fellow, what are you doing?

A: I want to put an end to my life.

B: Are you joking? Please, come down from there.

A: Nobody can do anything for me any more.

C (*Entering*): Hey! What the hell is he doing?

A: First of all, don't approach me. I'll throw myself down, if you get near.

C: What? Are you joking?

A: I am speaking seriously. I am here, upon an 800-metre high bridge, do you think I am joking?

B: What are your problems, then?

A: There's no use telling them.

C: But you can tell them, unburden yourself, please do it . . .

A: I have a whole lot of problems. Life has not appreciated me, and I cannot appreciate life.

B (*Sitting*): My husband left me alone, with a nine-month-old big tummy. What shall I do, shall I also kill myself?

C (*Getting near to A*): Can I offer you a cigarette?

A: Don't approach, however! Just the time to smoke a cigarette . . . (*He takes the cigarette and lights it*)

C: No, no, I'll give you another one later. Life is beautiful: a cigarette, a pie . . . (*draws near a little*)

A: (*As a reaction to these words, tries to fling himself into the void*)

C (*Loudly*): Salvatò, if you throw yourself over, this woman will abort. A child will die because of you.

B (*Fakes labour pains*): Help me! Help me!

A: (*Climbs over and draws near to help her*)

APPLAUSE

'The suicide' is an extemporaneous improvisation[12] format that had great success in the group: perhaps because it faces the theme of death without mincing its words, which is a recurrent element in the addict's universe; or because it strongly sets the symbol of falling, joining charm and terror; finally, because it is a metaphor of the uselessness of the 'reasonable' attempts to save the would-be victim. None of the participants in the improvisations, apart from A, survives: the efforts to convince the suicide not to jump, based upon commonsense, are all failing, and the thrill of looking at people jumping into the void is granted to the audience. Even C's attempts to get to the companion with arguments of everyday life ('Life is beautiful: a cigarette, a pie . . .') are powerless before an existential determination ('Life has not appreciated me, and I cannot appreciate life'). The only element of novelty is represented by the pregnant woman, even if her verbal exhortations are useless as well and don't arouse empathy. On the other hand, A is so absorbed in his own problem that he cannot see the other's problem. A turning point comes when the gradual approach of C, who while giving a reassuring message tries to reach a position from which he can grab the suicide, is abruptly interrupted by A, who perceives the manoeuvre and acts the gesture of leaning out and just about to fall. At this point the situation comes to a head and C, abdicating the prudence and friendly attitude kept till now, strikes A with a cutting call to reality, and to individual responsibility for the others ('A child will die because of you'). It is interesting to notice that this is the only moment in which C calls A by his true name. This strengthens the aspect of the connection between dramatic reality and ordinary reality, between 'world' and world. A call to reality that is also a call to action: to save a child who is about to be born means to save a project that does not belong to himself but to the whole of humankind, like the project of someone returned from far away who wants to build a life here, upon this land. Without a word, A hastens to offer help.

Meeting with death and meeting with life, falling and getting up again, losing oneself and finding oneself again: these are symbols of risk and change that pervade the existence of the addict like the existence of each one of us and that, in the dramatic process, are voiced through the shared imagination within the 'as if' frame. Certainly, along the process it is possible to deal with specific difficulties connected with the affective area as those related to emotional expression and containment, but the symbolic level is what produces a deep sense of integration and belonging.

In one of the last sessions of an annual cycle, I suggested an imaginative game to the group focused on the use of the voice. The group members stand in a circle, they experience the various breathing positions (diaphragmatic, thoracic, pectoral) and they practise their voices through the perception of *resounders* and the visualization of images connected with the height of the sound. With the deep voice (or stomach voice), connected with diaphragmatic breathing, they have to imagine a flow of lukewarm water that fills the room flowing downward; with the middle voice (or chest voice), connected with thoracic breathing, a puff of wind travelling toward the world; with the high voice (or head voice), connected with pectoral breathing, a beam of light directed toward the sky. Breathing and voicing loosen the tensions and induce an intense concentration. Now the whole group closes their eyes and tunes up in unison a low note for a preset number of breathings. Then I ask them to continue to utter free sounds together. The vocalism lasts a few minutes. At the end, when eyes are opened again, I see smiles lighting up and intertwining, and a pleasant feeling of relaxation and comfort is unfolded within the group. At this point, I ask them to think about the images that crossed their minds during the improvisation, and to choose the more intriguing ones. The image selected is of a quiet mountain lake, on a moonlight night, above which the spirits of the dead flutter, and each one tells a story. M, who in the suicide game had been the first to die, says: 'I was a horse, a white, free and powerful horse. I ran and ran, happy, without ever getting tired. But I was alone, even when I was with the others, and I died of solitude. And now every night I still run along the lake, as once before, and I am a spirit. Let me run together with you.'

Chapter 7

Disabilities

Why should it not be possible, Ewald? What is forbidden to people able to use their legs, can happen to you: they go past many things, never stopping, and they run away in front of many others. You are destined by God, Ewald, to be a standstill in the middle of this whole fury. Don't you feel as everything stirs around you? The other people chase the days, and when at last they reach one, I am afraid that they cannot even speak to it. But you, my dear, simply sit by the window, and wait; and to him who waits something happens, sooner or later.

(Rainer Maria Rilke, *The Stories of Good Lord*, 1900)

A name and a place

I remember a primary school teacher (fortunately, not so many teachers are like that) who, complaining about the difficult circumstances of her work, referred to her class as composed of 'twenty-five children and a handicapped', using the term as a noun rather than an adjective. The term handicap has survived for almost two centuries within horse racing, before being used first in specialized language and later in common language to define, according to the Zingarelli dictionary, an 'incapability to provide by oneself, entirely or partially, the normal necessities of the individual and social life, determined by a deficiency, congenital or acquired, physics or psychic [. . .] and having individual, family and social consequences'. If life is a race, then many have as their lot some limitations that don't allow them to reach the finishing line. This associative thread fits well with a standpoint that recognizes the problem rather than the person, or identifies the person with the problem. In the English language, from which the term was born, the word handicap is no longer in use, as it evokes, rather than 'hand in cap' (which refers to an ancient game that nobody quite remembers any more), 'cap in hand', reminding us of the pathetic figures of afflicted people and beggars that, from the *Beggar's Opera* to Dickens, populated English literature.

It is quite the same with the term 'disabled', which has come back into use in recent years, as it is considered more 'elegant' than handicapped. But here we find a negative definition too: dis-abled is a person who doesn't know how to do things, who doesn't own abilities or attitudes that other people possess. *Homo abilis* is how we called our ancestor who first splintered stones to use them as tools (presumably to kill). *Homo sapiens* should have followed on his heels, but if we look at what the world is like, we might wonder whether he ever arrived. Somebody even tried to resolve the problem by making up a neologism – 'diversabled' – which has a lovely meaning but is so woolly and premeditated as to sound almost ridiculous.

Certainly the terms 'disabled' and 'handicapped' are softer and less violent than many of the awful and insulting epithets that were used beforehand, such as 'retarded' or 'subnormal'. The fact still remains that we have serious difficulties in thinking up a name for those people, as well as in thinking of a place for them. Until recent times, disabled people were still subjected to what Foucault called 'the great internment'. They were confined in institutes or charities, or even in insane asylums, forgotten by the world and rarely considered more than mere things. In Italy we have an excellent law that recognizes the rights of disabled people, coherent with one of the basic principles of modern democracy: the principle of equality.

Of course, to have a good law is not enough: we also need tools, funds and training. But above all we need a cultural horizon that allows us to include diversity in our experience of the world. This means reinventing our identity as open to difference rather than as a fortress to be defended. If differences frighten us, it is because they belong to us, because they remind us of our own limitations. We can deny them, but we cannot elude them: discarding differences is entropy and death. The dramatherapist Pat Brudenell has written:

> The confrontation of handicap, stirs within us the feelings of our own handicap. The discomfort, the pain, the immobility, the withdrawal of the autistic child, brings us face-to-face with the despair inside ourselves. At times the overwhelming sense of helplessness in that child cries out for us to help them. And what can we do?
>
> (in Jennings 1988: 185)

Approaching the difference with a mood of attention and thoughtfulness may place into crisis our balance – so arduously built and supported by the trust in our abilities – and present us with the undeniable proof of our finitude as human beings. Nevertheless, being also the sign of another world view and another possibility of existence, it leads to an enrichment.

The time of drama

To be able to gain this kind of approach, we need to suspend the time of our abilities and to put ourselves in a listening stance.

I cherish the memory of a scene I saw a few years ago. I was with my family, for a short holiday, in Cefalù, a fair Norman town that in summer turns into a Moloch of leisure time, an enormous factory of compulsory fun in which every place is a place of appearing, of obsessive pleasure hunting, of frantic excitement with no direction. While looking at that continuous whirling of people's heads, anxious to sip every single drop of the true life bestowed by the exaltation of the vacation, the verses of the great American poet Robinson Jeffers came to my mind:

> When the sun shouts and people abound
> One thinks there were the ages of the stone and the age of bronze,
> And the iron age; iron the unstable metal;
> Steel made of iron, unstable as his; the towered-up cities
> Will be stains of rust on mounds of plaster.
> Roots will not pierce the heaps for a time, kind rains will cure them
> Then nothing will remain of the iron age
> And of these people but a thigh bone or so, a poem
> Stuck in the world's thought, splinters of glass
> In the rubbish dump, a concrete dam far off in the mountains . . .
> (R. Jeffers, *Summer Holiday*, 1925)

Sitting at a table in a beach café at dusk, such thoughts crossed my mind. While I was looking at the 'ten thousand beings' that 'all together actively struggle',[1] with an incessant rhythm like an advertising spot or a video clip, my attention was drawn to a scene taking place at a table nearby. Three people were sitting there: two boys aged about twenty, one slim with long hair, and the other sturdier, with a short and thick black beard; and a blonde and slender girl in a wheelchair. All three kept silent, drinking something with a straw. The girl's gaze wandered over the outer scene: the people still lingering on the beach, those saying goodbye and arranging dates for the night, those getting into cars or onto mopeds to go and have fun somewhere else. She seemed, at first sight, rather melancholic, but every now and then she turned, not without some toil, toward her companions and, looking at them, she softly smiled. The boys rested their drinks for a while, and they smiled too. I don't know how long this scene lasted, but I can certainly say that it was happening in a different time than the time of the surrounding world, beaten with video clip pulsation. It was indeed a rarefied time in which something happened, a tiny ripple perhaps, but full of astonishing intensity and meaning, that involved me, who was only a spectator, in a deep experience of sharing. This is the time of drama. And it doesn't have anything to do with the time of abilities, neither with the *taylorism* of daily efficiency, nor with the frenzy of possession and consumption of things and people. In the time of drama, encounter is possible between different experiences of the world because, free from the limitations and the anxieties of racing, it can expand to hold and welcome the whole of them.

A flower in the cement

In the second meeting of the drama workshop, V tells a story: it is the story of a flower that cannot grow because someone has unloaded heavy blocks of cement all around it. 'People should not destroy nature,' concludes V with his jerky speech, underlining the ecological moral of the story. But we all immediately perceive that the image hides many deeper meanings, and we are involved in them, at different levels. In its simplicity that connects manifold universes of sense, meanwhile evoking them and setting them in a unique image at a high affective degree, the story is an 'open metaphor'; a poetic creation comparable to Eugenio Montale's 'Sunflower', to Blake's 'The Sick Rose' or to William Carlos Williams's 'The Crimson Cyclamen'. The therapist proposes to stage it as it is, without further working out. V chooses F as a protagonist, a girl nailed on a wheelchair like him, and like him keen on stories and poems. F is helped to go into the middle of the stage and all the other people set around her as blocks of cement. The scene is without words, but extraordinarily moving. In the middle of that throbbing stillness, F's many attempts to rise, made with an actual, intense physical effort, express the pain of her denied body, the weight of a threshold impossible to cross. They reach a mythical dimension, in which Sisyphus and Icarus loom up, reminding us of the pointlessness of human efforts and the eternal struggle between desire and limitation.

To all this drama is witness and mirror, and the sense of impotence evoked is reflected in the silence and immobility of all those bodies piled up one upon the other. I suggest they close their eyes and listen to their own feelings. After a couple of minutes when everybody keeps their eyes closed – the bodies in contact one with another, breath and blood flows interweaving a rhythmic counterpoint – a movement slowly begins, a slight oscillation that becomes little by little a wave that makes them swing together from side to side, so they look as if they are cradling each other. Someone has the idea to sing a lullaby and little by little the voices gently gather into a single voice: lullaby, lullaby, baby. . . Then, a great silence and a breath of peace. At the end of the scene, everybody gets up again. Those who need help easily find it and there are many smiles spreading around. It is a field of flowers that grows and opens, each one in its own way, each one in its own time.

The body has turned from a sign of restraint into a symbol of nourishment, growth and transformation. In drama, the body is accepted as it is, without the claim to educate it to efficiency – even though to a theatrical efficiency – but respected in its native particularity, telling a story and an identity that make it the starting point of a sharing process. Giulia Innocenti Malini, one of the main experts in Italy of social dramaturgy, has written:

> The disabled body engages some counterbalancing actions, which transform the experience, the intensity, the rhythm, the action, the equilibriums, the perceptions and the expression. They build new and unusual signs, languages and symbols. When theatre meets disability, it must set in a deep situation of listening and reciprocity. That is to say, to allow the otherness of this bodily condition to become the hinge of the expressive research, and by means of it, to transform and enrich itself.
>
> (in Badolato *et al.* 2000: 91)

If the body is not a mere organism, but an answer to the world, in drama the disabled people can afford to take unusual routes, pivoting not on what they don't know how to do or cannot do, as often happens in classical rehabilitation processes, but on new configurations that find sense and justification in the shared imagination of the group. But drama also outlines the frame of a meeting in which the mimetic flows can come into play once more:

> The dramatic process allows exploring and going along again those lines of the relational evolution of the body that could have been disowned during the developmental experience. The actor is par excellence a person who sets again in motion his polarities of separation and connection, developing and strengthening them. He

does it in the very moment in which he draws the circle of the theatre and he distinguishes within from without. Both, even connected, are separated.

(ibid.: 89)

The dramatherapist Anna Chesner, in *Dramatherapy for People with Learning Disabilities* (1995), which is perhaps the best book about using drama with disabled people, employs the fascinating metaphor of the tree to tell what Dramatherapy can do for these people. Body is related to the root of the tree, which Chesner relates to the theme of Solidity and with the element Earth. The bodywork allows building nonthematic bonds, founded upon trust and nourishment, upon the development and the reinforcement of the senses and of what Gardner (1983) calls bodily kinaesthetic intelligence. The trunk of the tree is related to the theme of Growth and the element Wood: the dynamic of spontaneity/rules, the emotional containment created by the game structure, opens the doors of the shared creative process. The branches of the tree are connected with the theme of Expansion and with the element Air: imagination and expression foster interpersonal abilities and the extension of the role potentialities. The leaves of the tree remind us of the theme of Transformation and the element Light: the change is produced by self-awareness and personal responsibility.

But the metaphor of the tree leads us further: to think of a path of growth, expansion and change that must be supported with gentleness and benevolence, with an absolute respect for the pace and the desires of the other, and above all with mimetic understanding and empathy. As Pat Brudenell reminds us:

Unless we can *believe* that we share a common ground, then the role of the therapist will be a redundant one.

(in Jennings 1988: 184)

Epilogue

As a closure, I would like to tell you one more tale: the story of my own first encounter with the transformative power of drama.

In the spring of 1979, the first year of the course at the Theatre School *Teatés* was in its closing stages. For me, like many others, it had been an extremely intense experience: led by unique teachers, we felt on the one hand like initiates undergoing a path of wisdom and on the other we were a little inebriated and dazed from the passion.

That spring was also for me an awfully critical moment: recovering from a recent love heartbreak, on bad terms with my parents, with a strong feeling of guilt for having disappointed them, I glimpsed many different routes in front of me, but each of them was shadowy and sown with doubts.

While in this confused and gloomy mood, I was refreshed by a visit, two days before the school's final performance, from Alberto, an old friend of mine, a person of profound learning and gifted with an inner wisdom. We did not talk about my issues; I often received the best advice through his silences. He and I, together with a group of environmentalists, had promoted a campaign to protect Monte Pellegrino, the holy mountain of Palermo, which was threatened by a weird 'tourist' project that included the building of a road halfway up the slope and a golf course on a plateau rich in Phoenician archaeological finds. We undertook many trips upon the mountain, following historical, naturalistic and ethnographic routes, but this time it was a special event: Alberto had succeeded in getting the keys to enter the Addaura caves, a Palaeolithic location of considerable importance with very famous graffiti. Although they have been systematically studied, nevertheless the graffiti are still puzzling. The most well-known one depicts a ritual dance. Some men with spears in their hands, wearing on their faces something that can seem like a bird beak or a pointed beard, move around two figures on the ground, whose arms are bent and perhaps tied with strings. Someone had interpreted the scene as a bloody sacrifice, comparing the image of the two people lying on the ground with the *incaprettamento* (capra = goat), a gruesome mafia practice; someone else saw it as a rite of passage, where the two people underwent a proof of courage. The graffiti are on a wall many metres high and you have to clamber up a narrow iron staircase and stand upon a little platform to see them from close up. Hanging in space, hanging in time, we stood silent for almost an hour to watch those finely painted figures dancing an ancient and mysterious dance, with their lithe bodies and their enigmatic bird masks.

Shortly after this outstanding experience, the time came for the school's final performance. The text chosen by my group was a fragment of a Harold Pinter play, *The Birthday*. The role I was given – as far as I can remember – was that of an Irishman, half-drunkard, slimy and servile but prone to violence, who supports the underhand manoeuvres of his master, directed towards the psychological destruction of the protagonist. In helping this despicable action, he seems almost unaware, completely tricked by the master's evil charm, to the point that he entirely loses his own identity, which peeps out occasionally in his homeland memories.

Submissive, violent, foolish and debauched: I felt every one of these features so far from me, or at least from what I longed to be, but they emerged sometimes as scorching self-accusations in my depressive moments, which were rather recurrent at that time.

The performance was successful, yet what gave me a profound sense of wholeness was not the applause (after all, it was a friendly audience consisting of my own schoolmates) but the sensation of being on the one hand in a sort of trance, within which I could let the character seize me, in a certain sense contaminate me, highlighting ruthlessly and shamelessly some features I considered dreadful, and which I was authorized then to pull out as *theirs*, not mine; on the other hand, I could give myself permission to laugh about them, to make a caricature of them, therefore keeping my distance from them. It was a catharsis in an Aristotelian sense: in some ways I was purifying myself, setting myself free from those stinking miasma that poisoned my soul; I had the chance to make them alive and visible through the other, the character, and to lay them down as I dropped it, taking off the mask. But the most stunning sensation was that, after all, what I was doing was not unlike what the Addaura dancers were doing, many millenniums ago and just now: to exorcise violence and death through the Form. That was a moment of enlightenment. Shortly after I met my future wife and a new adventure could start: I was beginning to become adult.

Theatre, as Richard Courtney maintains, is but the tip of the iceberg of something larger, a quality deeply rooted in human nature: the potentiality of being 'as if', a quality expressed in child play, in ritual and in various forms of theatre. Courtney calls *Drama* this quality, describing it as *re-cognition*; Richard Schechner calls it *Performance*, and defines it as *restored behaviour*. Though seemingly conflicting, what these definitions have in common is the principle that people own the potential to confer meaning to their experience of the world and to transform it, reworking it creatively through imagination. This is Dramatherapy's root hypothesis.

My work over the past ten years has been devoted to experiment with this hypothesis and to deepen it: the book you are just finishing is a testimony to this research. Above all what I hope to transmit is the feeling that Dramatherapy is neither just a technique, nor a method, but a living body, with a mind (the theories, the empiric knowledge and the beliefs), a heart (the art of the encounter) and a spine (that is ourselves as persons, witnesses and sources of an inexhaustible energy of creation and transformation).

Afterword

How far that little candle throws his beams!
So shines a good deed in a naughty world.
(Shakespeare, *The Merchant of Venice*,
V, I, 91–92)

And so shines this remarkable book in a world that is volatile, changing and chaotic. Salvo Pitruzzella has achieved something quite remarkable in bringing a fresh experience to this elusive world that makes up theatre, drama and Dramatherapy. He speaks from a bedrock of solid theatre experience and research, and uses it as a lens to focus on the pathways of healing that Dramatherapy can provide.

The detailed development of 'dramatic reality' in Patterns of Drama is a crucial concept for Dramatherapy. The journey that the actor or client makes from the everyday reality of the world, to the dramatic reality of the 'world' and then back again is a process of supreme importance and complexity. It is essentially a human phenomenon and necessary for maturation. Many people cannot differentiate the two realities of their experience and all merges into one. We can see this very obviously in the play of toddlers where imagination and life are not always separated. When my granddaughter Mary told me that the car had got scratched because a monster was trying to get inside, rather than the everyday fact that her mother has scraped the car on a gatepost, she illustrates this very point. Eventually the child is able to move in and out of the two realities appropriately.

People with mental ill health often lose the borders between the two states, more easily understood by the idea of losing the capacity to react or even act in the 'as if' mode. People who are psychotic in one sense are trapped in dramatic reality as they have lost the capacity to move into the everyday. Similarly some psychopathic personalities could be described as being locked into everyday reality. Their imagination is the lived reality of their everyday experience. This has enormous implications because, for example, people are killed for real rather than in dramatic action. The efficacy of Dramatherapy as a healing medium is only just beginning to be explored or rediscovered.

There is one aspect of our 'being in the world' that I would like readers of this book to think about. Whereas we are beginning to understand the dramatic processes through the body, the mask, the game, and the story, as Salvo so lucidly demonstrates, we have not yet put these into the wider global context. We have not yet developed an ecological model of Dramatherapy (or even theatre) where we can look at the relationship between nature and culture; where we can look at a nature-centred world rather than a person-centred world. Eventually we shall experience nature firsthand and not just through the lens of culture.

This book can be described by Titania's imagery, where she talks about the disruption in the natural and the human worlds being caused by dissent in the fairy and spiritual worlds. We live in a world of rivalry, competitiveness and warmongering and this book is about a peace process through the therapeutic experience of the drama. This process is not just for our clients, it is for all of us, and it is about us all living together in greater understanding with our environment.

I want to read this book again – and again. Thank you Salvo for a jewel in the cave.

Sue Emmy Jennings
Glastonbury, UK

Appendix:
Observation grids

Group observation grid

1. GENERAL DATA

Context ....
....

Date .... Time .... Session n .... of a cycle of ....
Participants:
Clients...
....
....

Workers ....
....
....

Structural notes ....
....
....

2. SETTING UP

Preliminary Considerations ....
....
....
....
....
....
....
....

Hypotheses for the session:
Foundation ....

....

....

Creation ....

....

....

....

Sharing ....

....

....

....

3. SESSION REPORT

Group mood: ....

....

....

....

Session description:
Foundation ....

....

....

....

Creation ....

....

....

....

Sharing ....

....

....

Meaningful contents: ....

....

....

....

....

....

....

Problems: ....

....

....

....

....

Hypotheses for the next session: ....

....

....

....

....

Individual observation grid

Name ....

Date .... Time...

Session n .... Of a cycle of ....

	Interaction	

Coming into play

☐ Destructive   ☐ Withdrawn   ☐ Shyly participative

☐ Active   ☐ Protagonist

Give/take

☐ Doesn't offer nor accepts cues   ☐ Accepts/no offer

☐ Offers/no acceptation   ☐ Both offers and accepts

Collaboration

☐ No collaboration   ☐ Follows the instructions

☐ Discusses the instructions

☐ Creatively works out the instructions

☐ Suggests ideas   ☐ Proposes structures

Comments: ....

....

....

Notes: ....

....

....

	Role	

Definition ....
....

Quality ....
....

Function ....
....

Style ....
....

Landy's Taxonomy Reference ....
....

Choosing modes:

☐ Casual   ☐ Group transaction

☐ Choice (protagonist)   ☐ Assigned by a protagonist

☐ Assigned by the therapist   ☐ Individual Improvisation

Focus:

☐ Constant   ☐ Fluctuating   ☐ Superficial   ☐ Absent

Distance:

☐ Whole performance   ☐ Only verbal performance

☐ Playing himself/herself with little variations

☐ Playing himself/herself

Complexity:

☐ Developed   ☐ Suitable
☐ Incomplete   ☐ Incoherent

Comments: ....
....
....
....

Notes: ....
....
....
....
....
....

Notes

Introduction: A healing theatre

1   William Blake, *The Marriage of Heaven and Hell.*
2   Some particularly important experiences were fruitful, producing respectful or rebellious sons, imitators, disciples and heretics. Among these teachers, we must remember the Americans: Richard Schechner, Julian Beck, Peter Schumann, who shouted 'from the heart of the beast'. Surprisingly, from dismal communist Poland the genius of Grotowski sparkled, and continued to influence strongly theatrical research to the end of the millennium with his numerous descendants. Perhaps the most important is Eugenio Barba who, with his other filiations, programmatically recovers the anthropological aspect of Artaud's thought, seeking the ritual essence of theatre in the encounter with cultural otherness.
3   I cherish a memory, for instance, of the political rituals of the Living Theatre, that succeeded in involving hundreds of people – even simple passers-by – in events of absolute ethical tension.
4   Here as well the greatest masters are from the Anglo-Saxon world: Viola Spolin and Keith Johnstone. Though their backgrounds are different (the former a teacher, the latter a theatre director), they developed models and techniques which are to a large extent complementary. Even if Improvisation is aimed primarily at theatre performances, its applications in social and educational fields are worthy of note, as is the case with Spolin's work in schools (see Spolin 1986). Also worthy of mention is the work of Daniel Wiener (see Wiener 1994), who uses Johnstone's techniques from a therapeutic viewpoint in family therapy.
5   The first seeds have been planted by Peter Slade: the word Dramatherapy first appeared printed in his works in 1959, though his practical work and his research on Dramatherapy had started long before. He was the first person to speak on this at the British Medical Association before World War II. His teachings are still influential today. The development of Dramatherapy as an art of healing is undoubtedly tied with the name of Sue Jennings. She definitely crossed the border between theatre supporting therapy and a renewed dramatic art, springing anew in every group, healing as creative. The main ideas underlying my own practice of Dramatherapy are drawn from their example, as well as from Roger Grainger's and Robert Landy's

contributions. (For a concise history of Dramatherapy in Britain, see Jennings 1995c; in the USA, where it is called Drama Therapy, see Lewis and Johnson 2000).

6   We must not forget that tragedy was much more than an artistic product in the sense in which we intend it today; it was a collective event with a strong social value.

7   Υποϰϱιτής, from which is derived the term 'hypocrite'.

I Person

1   Actually, the curtain of the opera opens on Don Giovanni running away. The scene that we are talking about is therefore only imagined.

2   Giovanni Falcone and Paolo Borsellino, both killed by the *Mafia* in 1992 in two war-like attacks, are still the symbols of the resistance of Sicilian people against this aged tyranny.

3   It must be noted that the void of Buddhism is not to be understood in the usual sense (as an absence of objects). It is rather a void/full, whose metaphor, in the mystical development of Buddhism, is 'Pure Light'. However, the oriental conceptions of the world have never given great importance to the 'to be/not to be' dichotomy that from Parmenides to Hamlet has tormented Western thought.

2 Threshold

1   'The sphere of the inter-human extends far beyond that of sympathy. Banal situations can belong to it, such as the exchange of glances between two strangers in a tram, who conveniently choose not to meet each other. But one must also include all the encounters among adversaries, however secondary they may be, if they influence the mutual attitude; if, that is, something happens between them, even though in the most imperceptible way. It doesn't matter that at that time the accent is placed more or less on feelings. The important thing is that between two people, each one experiences the other as a determined other, that both perceive the other equally [. . .] This is the decisive thing: not to be considered as an object' (Buber 1925: 297).

2   To continue our discourse on imagination we must take into consideration the work of the artist who, more than any other, put this faculty at the centre of his vision of the world and of art, William Blake (1757–1827).

3   For a thorough study of Imagination doctrine in Blake, compared with philosophy of his time, see Frye (1947); Paley (1970). See also the remarkable Kathleen Raine's conference about *Science and Imagination in W.B.* in Raine (1991).

3 Elements

1   Campbell's investigation is mostly centred in literature, identifying in two masterpieces of the nineteenth century, James Joyce's *Ulysses* and Thomas Mann's *The Enchanted Mountain*, the greatest expression of the modern age individual myth, in its relationship with ancient and deep symbols and imaginary structures; but he also finds this mythical individual/universal

connection in Picasso's art and in the work of such poets as W. B. Yeats, T. S. Eliot and Robinson Jeffers.

2 At the time of writing these tiny Japanese mutant monsters are the heroes of the moment. Probably, given the ephemeral permanence of these phenomena, when you read this book nobody would remember who or what they were.

3 See the form/process dynamics in Bateson (1979).

4 In Pitruzzella (2000).

5 'Your children are not your children./ They are the sons and daughters of Life's longing for itself./ They come through you but not from you,/ And though they are with you yet they belong not to you.' K. Gibran, *The Prophet*.

6 When stories travel, in oral transmission, they often move toward the centre of the continuum. Examples of this are the so-called urban legends (see Brunvand 1987); stories that are spread, often across the continents, and are told from time to time as testimonies, but are actually inventions. However, even in historiography, which among the forms of narration is the one that most aspires to 'the truth', the importance of the points of view, of the ideologies, of the biases, of the deliberate mystifications through the trans-formation of 'what really happened' in an acceptable account, is quite clear. For example, it is not long since we began to consider the events of European colonial expansion from the point of view of the vanquished. The stories of the extermination of the American Indians, for instance, throw a different light on the history of the United States, revealing how the foundation of a nation, for long seen as the country of freedom and democracy, is stained with the tears and blood of innocent people (see Brown 1970).

7 When a story becomes everybody's story, when the teller gives a part of himself to the world and the world thanks him, it becomes possible for everybody to mirror themselves in it. For millennia people have told fairytales. Italo Calvino, who explored at length the universe of fairytales to compose his monumental work, believed that the fairytales are 'the catalogue of the destinies that can be given to a man and to a woman, especially for the part of life that exactly is the making of a destiny: the youth, from the birth that often brings itself an auspice or a sentence, to the departure from home, to the trials of becoming adult and then mature, so confirming themselves as human beings' (Calvino 1956: xv). But the mirroring into fairytales does not occur only at the resonance level of the structures of human life's development in the social world; it expands toward a level that goes beyond everyday awareness, toward the universe of symbols. Kings, queens, princes and beggars, magicians, witches and elves animate the world in which gods once dwelled. It is not an accident that ancient mythological motives can be found in traditional Western fairytales. Just like play, even the fairytale is threatened by cultural standardization. When Calvino compiled his book, in the 1950s, drawing most on eighteenth-century folklorists' transcriptions, the oral tradition of the fairytale was already dying. Today, with the dreadful development of the mass media, which roughly colonized all other forms of communication, the knowledge of fairytales passes through books (and also through the internet where there are many websites devoted to fairytales and other traditional stories). Paradoxically, just in the last 50 years the deep developmental value of

fairytales has been underlined by psychologists and educators, just as the importance of the other cultures has been rediscovered by anthropologists in the very moment in which these cultures were about to be destroyed. The fact remains that many elements of fairytales, both in structure and content, are immediately comprehensible, I would say recognizable, even by those who have never listened to them. This makes me think that it is true that, as Joseph Campbell stated, 'fairy tales are the primer of the figured language of the soul'.

8   It is worth noting that the last name of Fernando Pessoa, the Portuguese poet who wrote his works as if they were written by various different individuals, means 'person'.

9   The Taoist text *Chuang-Tzu* contains the following tale:
Chuang-Tzu and Hui-Tzu walked on the dike of the river Hao.
'Little fishes come out for swimming at their liking,' Chuang-Tzu said. This is their happiness.
'You are not a fish,' Hui-Tzu objected. 'How do you know the happiness of the fishes?'
'You are not me,' Chuang-Tzu replied. 'How do you know that I don't know the happiness of the fishes?'
'I am not you,' Hui-Tzu insisted, 'and certainly I don't know you, but certainly you are not a fish: the conclusion is that you don't know the happiness of the fishes.'
'Please consider the original question,' Chuang-Tzu said. 'You have said: "How do you know the happiness of the fishes?" You have asked because you knew that I knew. I have known it on this river Hao.'

4 Structures

1   My psychodramatist friends will forgive me for this assonance with 'Morel's invention', a novel by A. Bioy Casares (1940), which is the story of a machine that, every day at the same time, materializes always the same scene recorded a long time ago – a challenge to death through the repetition (which is exactly the opposite of the vitality and of the spontaneity advocated by Moreno).

2   'During a session of impromptu theatre, a young actress, playing a *different* fact, finds herself transformed by the cathartic action of the role she is taking on (a murdered prostitute) and the relationship with her husband is improved' (Schützenberger 1970: 244).

3   'The complex of feelings that attract or reject a person, born from the characteristics perceived in the other person, is called *tele*. [. . .] In a *tele* relationship, people can communicate among themselves 'at a distance', be in contact 'from far' and send some messages 'at the feeling level' (Boria 1983: 29).

4   Moreno writes: 'Since its origins the premises of scientific medicine have been that the centre of the physical distress is the individual organism. Then, the treatment is applied to the centre of distress designated by the diagnosis. [. . .] When the newborn psychiatry began to use scientific methods, the axioms of physical diagnoses and treatment were also applied automatically to mental troubles. [. . .] The change of the locus of the therapy literally

means a revolution in what has always been considered correct medical practice' (Moreno 1946: 379–80).

5 The categories listed by Yalom are as follows: 1. Information. 2. Hope infusion. 3. Universality. 4. Altruism. 5. Corrective recapitulation of the family primary group. 6. Development of techniques of socialization. 7. Imitative behaviour. 8. Interpersonal learning. 9. Group cohesion. 10. Catharsis. The list is not in order of importance, neither rigidly prescriptive: they are rather 'interdependent: they never come nor operate separately' (1970: 19).

6 'The games emerged out of necessity. I didn't sit at home and dream them up. When I had a problem, I made up a game. When another problem came up, I just made up a new game' (Interview, *Los Angeles Times*, 26 May 1974).

7 In Johnstone's version of this game, it has a didactic finality: it is therefore preceded by a phase in which the giver has the responsibility of the gift. Then the trainer stops the game and suggests new rules, according to which the invention of the object is charged to the receiver. 'An important change of thinking is involved here. When the actor concentrates on making the thing he *gives* interesting, every actor seems in competition, and feels it. When they concentrate on making the gift they *receive* interesting, then they generate warmth between them' (Johnstone, 1979: 101).

8 I am in debt for this exercise to my friend and teacher Marco Baliani.

9 It is nearly the same range of activity that Caillois includes under the category of the play, setting them on the axle of the polarity between *paideia* and *ludus* therefore in regard to the relationship with the rules.

10 A tool that I have found very useful in this phase is the 6PSM (Six pieces story-making) by Moholi Lahad (1992, 2000), whose aim is to ascertain which are people's favourite strategies for coping with the stress. The subject is asked to develop a story from a six-part structure (which is a very synthetic version of Propp's functions). The story is then analysed with a grid based on a model that Lahad calls BASICPh (acronym for Beliefs and values, Affective, Social, Imaginative, Cognitive, Physical), which identifies the different areas of the personality in which the coping resources are placed.

11 See Pitruzzella 2002.

12 Among the most interesting ones, besides the already quoted Arieti, see Bruner (1964); De Bono (1967, 1970). For a detailed and complete research into the concept of creativity in the psychological area, see Carotenuto (1991). For a sociological approach, see Melucci (1994).

13 The verse is in various poems. In 'Vala or the four Zoas' we read: 'Arise you little glancing wings & sing your infant joy/ Arise & drink your bliss/ For every thing that lives is holy for the source of life/ Descends to be a weeping babe/ For the Earthworm renews the moisture of the sandy plain.'

14 'Although human beings seek balance and integration, they live in a world of conflicting psychological and social forces that often lead to imbalance and separation. [...] At some hypothetical midpoint, people have the potential to find effective ways to live within and among their roles while accepting the contradictory pulls of competing personae. *Like accomplished jugglers with just the right number of balls in the air, they move forward,*

aware that if they take their precarious state of balance for granted, their balls will tumble to the ground (Landy 1993: 14, my italics).

15 For an in-depth discussion about supervision in Dramatherapy, see Tselikas-Portmann (1999); Lahad (2000).

16 This is an elaboration of an exercise suggested by Sue Jennings (1998), with the interpolation of a creative writing exercise devised by Keith Johnstone (1999).

5 Mental health

1 William Cowper (1731–1800) was a fine poet of English early romanticism. Gifted with an exceptional sensibility joined with a deep psychological frailty, he led a solitary and troubled existence, marked by long stays in the insane asylum. Blake, who had a high regard for Cowper (and who himself had been considered mad), was commended to illustrate a poet's life, but the portrait he made of Cowper was refused by the publisher and by his heirs because it was considered 'horrible and dreadful' for it expressed too much folly. In the quoted comment, Blake probably refers to a vision.

2 Exceptions to this are the autobiographic testimonies of 'learned' mad people (see Porter 1987).

3 'Madness becomes a form related to reason, or rather madness and reason eternally enter a reversing relationship, producing the fact that every madness has its reason that judges and dominates it, and every reason has its madness in which it finds its derisive truth' (Foucault 1963: 47).

4 The systematic destruction of in-patients' personal identities that occurred in many insane asylums is testified by the fact that they lost name and story upon entering the institution. They could not hold personal objects that tied them to their own past and were often renamed with nicknames. Maria Fuxa, a Sicilian poetess who has spent a long part of her life confined in the psychiatric hospital of Palermo, writes of a companion: 'Picchì bùmmula mi chiamanu,/ ridennu e satannu, comu li sguaiati./ Ma iu gridu cu tutti li me forzi:/ Fernanda mi chiamu, e beddu è lu me nomu! [They call me 'jar', laughing and jumping, with coarse words. But I shout with all of my strengths: Fernanda is my name, and beautiful my name is!] (*Voice of the Voiceless*, 1980).

5 In 1959 R. D. Laing's *The Divided Self* is published. In 1961 Goffman's book; in 1963 Foucault's *History of Madness in the Classical Age*; in 1964 Peter Brook stages Peter Weiss's *Marat-Sade*. In the same years, Franco Basaglia's early experiences took place in Gorizia.

6 We have to add that, despite the good intentions, the transformation is far from being complete, tied up as it is to independent fluctuations that go from the general zeitgeist of the society, to the dominant political orientations, to the pressures of the lobbies of the pharmaceutical industry, to the rivalries among professional guilds, to the frequent bad management of the health and social services.

7 What is rarely used in Dramatherapy within this context is the psycho-dramatic technique called *Double* – consisting of placing side by side or behind the actor's back (the protagonist, in the case of psychodrama) a person (usually the therapist) or more than one, giving voice to the character's inner

feelings – as it has the tendency to produce interpretations that might not be accepted or acknowledged by the subjects, or may condition in a captious way their free research.

8 On the polarity of feedback/calibration in the learning processes, see Bateson (1979: 258–68).

9 This is the part of Moreno's complex model that gave rise to many applications of 'role playing' in both the therapeutic and educational fields.

6 Addictions

1 G. Jervis has written upon the difference between habit and addiction: 'We speak of habituation to the toxic substance when the subject, besides introducing permanently in his own habits the toxic substance, is psychologically conditioned to its use to the point not succeeding without difficulty in performing without it his own daily activities. Addiction means that the organism of the subject inserted the toxic substance in his own metabolism, to the point of requiring an ever greater dose of it and showing troubles, withdrawal symptoms, if he is suddenly deprived of it' (Jervis 1975: 342).

2 I write these pages a few weeks after the tragic events of September 11 2001, when America and Europe discover the immense opium fields in Afghanistan, managed directly by terrorist groups.

3 'Heroin. And she is my wife, and she is my life,' sang Lou Reed. The Rolling Stones sang in praise of 'Brown Sugar' ('Brown Sugar, how come you taste so good/Brown Sugar, just like a young girl should'), or more explicitly they invoked 'Sister Morphine': 'Please, Sister Morphine, turn my nightmares into dreams.'

4 In 1978, in Cinisi, a seaside village near Palermo airport, the mafia brutally murdered Peppino Impastato, who opposed the extension of the airport and reported the new affairs of the mafia in the drug business. In the same years and in the same area, the first great heroin refineries were born in Sicily.

5 'The *flash*. It is a real explosion that invades body and mind, in a way comparable to orgasm. The experience of the flash is so fantastic that its memory will continually be recalled and searched for the following occasions' (Marcelli and Braconnier 1983: 307–8).

6 'The *planet*. Often compared to a shell of lukewarm water, the planet has two important characteristics that are not often described: it has a role of selective filter that attenuates any disagreeable feeling and allows only pleasant feelings to pass; it has in itself a rich content in terms of fantasy liberation; while it lasts, everything is permitted and everything can be dared' (ibid.: 307–8).

7 'The *descent*. It is a phase experienced and suffered. Little by little, the subject re-enters real life not only at bodily level (that is the withdrawal syndrome, or 'cold turkey') but also at psychic level. From a cosmic and fantastic world the subject returns to his everyday personal world. [. . .] To accept this situation seems intolerable to the subject, all the more because there is the memory, unfortunately made immediately attractive, accessible and realizable with a new puncture, at least as much he believes or hopes' (ibid.: 308).

8   'To be one of a crowd exempts a man from the consciousness of being an isolated self and takes him down into a kingdom less than personal, where there is no responsibility, where there is no right or wrong, neither need to think, nor to judge or to discern; there is only a strong and vague sense of communion, a shared excitement, a collective alienation. And this alienation is both more prolonged and less fatiguing than the one induced by the debauchery; the morning after is less depressing than the one following the self-poisoning with alcohol or morphine' (Huxley 1952: 310).

9   'As drunkenness, elementary sexuality, enjoyed for itself, and separated by the love, was once a god, beloved not only as the principle of fertility, but as demonstration of the immanent radical difference in every human being. [. . .] There is an elementary sexuality which is innocent and an elementary sexuality morally and aesthetically bleak. D. H. Lawrence has written in a very beautiful way of the former; Jean Genêt, with dreadful power and in detail, of the latter. The sexuality of Eden and the sexuality of the cesspit: both have the power to transport the individual beyond the limits of his isolated self. But the second and unfortunately more common variety transports those people surrendering to it to a lower plane of humanity, evokes the conscience and leaves the memory of a more complete alienation, rather than the first one' (ibid.: 309).

10 And it seems to me that the various attempts to unite social interventions with medical and psychological go in this direction.

11 See, among the others, Warren (1981); Dayton (1990); Boal (1992); Atkins (1994); Emunah (1994); Schotz (1998); Alschitz (1998).

12 Improvisations in Dramatherapy are classified as: *Planned improvisation*, when the essential parameters of the dramatic action (Who, Where, What) are entirely agreed in advance; *Extemporaneous improvisation*, when they are only partially agreed (for instance, we know the context and the characters, or at least their mutual roles in that determined situation, but the carrying out of the action – the plot – is left to improvisation); *Impromptu improvisation*, when only one or even none of the parameters is previously established (see Emunah 1994).

7 Disabilities

1   Tao Te Ching, XVI.

Bibliography

Alschitz, J. (1998) *La grammatical dell'attore*, Milano: Ubulibri.

American Psychiatric Association (1997) *DSM IV, Manuale Diagnostico e Statistico dei Disturbi Mentali*, Milano: Masson.

Ancelin Schutzenberger, A. (1970) *Lo psicodramma*, Firenze: Martinelli, 1972.

Anzieu, D. (1956) *Lo psicodramma analitico*, Roma: Astrolabio, 1979.

Arieti, S. (a cura di) (1959–66) *Manuale di psichiatria*, Torino: Boringhieri, 1969–70.

—— (1976) *Creatività. La sintesi magica*, Roma: Il Pensiero Scientifico Editore, 1979.

Aristotele (1987) *La poetica*, Firenze: La Nuova Italia.

Artaud, A. (1964) *Il teatro e il suo doppio*, Torino: Einaudi, 1968.

Atkins, G. (1994) *Improv!*, Portsmouth, NH: Heinemann.

Bachelard, G. (1960) *La poetica della rêverie*, Bari: Dedalo, 1972.

Badolato, G., Innocenti Malini, G., Fiaschini, F. and Villa, R. (2000) *La scena rubata. Appunti sull'handicap e il teatro*, Milano: Euresis.

Bailey, S. D. (1993) *Wings to Fly. Bringing Theatre Arts to Students with Special Needs*, Rockville, MD: Woodbine House.

Barba, E. (1993) *La canoa di carta*. Bologna: Il Mulino.

Barker, C. (1977) *Giochi di teatro*, Roma: Bulzoni, 2000.

Bateson, G. (1972) *Verso un'ecologia della mente*, Milano: Adelphi, 1976.

—— (1979) *Mente e Natura*, Milano: Adelphi, 1984.

Bateson, G. and Bateson, M. C. (1987) *Dove gli angeli esitano*, Milano: Adelphi, 1989.

Bateson, G. et. al. (1956) *'Questo è un gioco'*, Milano: Cortina, 1996.

Bergson, H. (1907) *L'evoluzione creatrice*, Bari: Laterza, 1957.

Bernardi, C., Cuminetti, B. and Dalla Palma, S. (a cura di) (2000) *I fuoriscena. Esperienze e riflessioni sulla drammaturgia nel sociale*, Milano: Euresis.

Bettelheim, B. (1977) *Il mondo incantato*, Milano: Feltrinelli, 1986.

Bhagavad Gita (1976), a cura di R. Gnoli, Torino: UTET.

Bianconi, R. A. (1999) *Ritualità nuziale nell'antica Roma*, Messina: Il Gabbiano.

Binswanger, L. (1921–1941) *Per un'antropologia fenomenologica*, Milano: Feltrinelli, 1970.

Biondi, M., Costantini, A. and Grassi L. (1995) *La mente e il cancro*, Roma: Il Pensiero Scientifico Editore.

Blatner, A. and A. (1988) *The Art of Play*. *Helping Adults Reclaim Imagination and Spontaneity*, New York: Brunner/Mazel, 1997.

Boal, A. (1974) *Il teatro degli oppressi*, Milano: Feltrinelli, 1977.

—— (1992) *Il poliziotto e la maschera*, Molfetta: La Meridiana, 1993.

Boella, L. and Buttarelli, A. (2000) *Per amore di altro*. *L'empatia a partire da Edith Stein*, Milano: Cortina.

Borges, J. L. (1960) 'L'artefice', in *Tutte le opere*, Milano: Mondadori, 1984.

Boria, G. (1983) *Tele*. *Manuale di psicodramma classico*, Milano: Franco Angeli.

Bowlby, J. (1969) *L'attaccamento alla madre*, Torino: Boringhieri, 1972.

—— (1973) *La separazione dalla madre*, Torino: Boringhieri, 1975.

—— (1975) *La perdita della madre*, Torino: Boringhieri, 1976.

—— (1988) *Una base sicura*, Milano: Cortina.

Brecht, B. (1957) *Scritti teatrali*, Torino: Einaudi, 1962.

Brecht, S. (1974) *Nuovo teatro americano. 1968–1973*, Roma: Bulzoni.

Brook, P. (1968) *The Empty Space*, Harmondsworth: Penguin.

—— (1993) *La porta aperta*, Milano: Anabasi, 1994.

Brown, D. (1970) *Seppellite il mio cuore a Wounded Knee*, Milano: Mondadori, 1972.

Bruner, J. (1964) *Il conoscere. Saggi per la mano sinistra*, Roma: Armando, 1968.

—— (1988) *La mente a più dimensioni*, Roma-Bari: Laterza.

Brunvand, J. H. (1987) *Leggende metropolitane*. *Storie improbabili raccontate come vere*, Genova: Costa & Nolan.

Buber, M. (1925) *Il principio dialogico*, Cinisello Balsamo: San Paolo, 1993.

Caillois, R. (1967) *I giochi e gli uomini. La maschera e la vertigine*, Milano: Bompiani, 1981.

Calvino, I. (1956) *Fiabe italiane*, Torino: Einaudi.

Calvino, I. (1960) *I nostri antenati*, Torino: Einaudi.

Campbell, J. (1949) *L'eroe dai mille volti*, Parma: Guanda, 2000.

—— (1959/1969) *Le maschere di dio*, Milano: Mondadori, 1990/1992.

—— (1969) *Il volo dell'anitra selvatica*, Milano: Mondadori, 1994.

Carotenuto, A. (1991) *Trattato di psicologia della personalità*, Milano: Cortina.

Carotenuto, A. (a cura di) (1992) *Trattato di psicologia analitica. Vol II: La dimensione clinica*, Torino: UTET.

Carrière, J.-C. (1998) *Il circolo dei contastorie*, Milano: Garzanti.

Caruso, S. and Kosoff, S. (1998) *The Young Actor's Book of Improvisation*, Portsmouth: Heinemann.

Cassady, M. (1993) *Acting Games. Improvisations and Exercises*, Colorado Springs: Meriwether.

Cattanach, A. (1999) *Process in the Arts Therapies*, London: Jessica Kingsley.

Chesner, A. (1995) *Dramatherapy for People with Learning Disabilities*, London: Jessica Kingsley.

Clifford, S. and Herrmann, A. (1999) *Making a Leap. Theatre of Empowerment*, London: Jessica Kingsley.

Coleridge, S. T. (1817) *Biographia Literaria*, Roma: Editori Riuniti, 1992.

Cooper, D. (a cura di) (1968) *Dialettiche della liberazione*, Torino: Einaudi.

Cox, M. (ed.) (1982) *Shakespeare Comes to Broadmoor*, London: Jessica Kingsley.

Cox, M. and Theilgaard, A. (1987) *Mutative Metaphors in Psychotherapy. The Eolian Mode*, London: Tavistock.

—— (1994) *Shakespeare as Prompter. The Amending Imagination and the Therapeutic Process*, London: Jessica Kingsley.

Cummings, E. E. (1965) *Fairy Tales*, San Diego: Voyager Books.

Dalla Palma, S. (2001) *Il teatro e gli orizzonti del sacro*, Milano: Vita e Pensiero.

Daniélou, A. (1992) *Miti e déi dell'India*, Como: RED, 1996.

Dayton, T. (1990) *Drama Games*, Deerfield Beach: Health Communications.

De Bono, E. (1967) *Il pensiero laterale*, Milano: Rizzoli, 1969.

—— (1970) *Creatività e pensiero laterale*, Milano: Rizzoli, 1998.

De Marinis, M. (1988) *Capire il teatro*, Firenze: La Casa Usher, 1997.

—— (2000) *In cerca dell'attore*, Roma: Bulzoni.

Demetrio, D. (1996) *Raccontarsi. L'autobiografia come cura di sé*, Milano: Cortina.

—— (1997) *Il gioco della vita. Kit autobiografico*, Milano: Guerini e associati.

Deriu, F. (1999) 'Lo spettro ampio delle attività performative', in R. Schechner (1977/1993) *Magnitudini della performance*, Rome: Bulzoni.

Di Bernardi, V. (1989) *Mahābhārata. L'epica indiana e lo spettacolo di Peter Brook*, Roma: Bulzoni.

Diderot, D. (1830) *Paradosso sull'attore*, Roma: Editori Riuniti, 1972.

Dumoulié, C. (1996) *Antonin Artaud*, Genova-Milano: Costa & Nolan, 1998.

Eakin, P. J. (1999) *How Our Lives Become Stories: Making Selves*, Ithaca: Cornell University Press.

Eliade, M. (1975) *Storia delle idee e delle credenze religiose*, Firenze: Sansoni, 1979.

Emunah, R. (1994) *Acting for Real*, New York: Brunner/Mazel.

—— (1995) 'From adolescent trauma to adolescent drama: group drama therapy with emotionally disturbed youth', in S. Jennings (ed.) *Dramatherapy with Children and Adolescents*, London: Routledge.

Erikson, E. H. (1968) *Gioventù e crisi d'identità*, Roma: Armando, 1974.

Falcone, G. (1991) *Cose di cosa nostra*, Milano: Rizzoli.

Feiffer, J. (1968) *Il trapianto del trauma*, Milano: Bompiani.

Fletcher, A. (1904) *Il rito Hako*, Firenze: La Nuova Italia, 1970.

Foster Damon, S. (1965) *A Blake Dictionary*, Hanover: University Press of New England, 1988.

Foucault, M. (1963) *Storia della follia nell'età classica*, Milano: Rizzoli, 1976.

Fox, J. (1986) *Acts of service*, New Paltz: Tusitala, 1994.

Frye, N. (1947) *Fearful Symmetry. A Study of William Blake*, Princeton: Princeton University Press.

Fuxa, M. (1980) *Voce dei senza voce*, Palermo: ASLA.

Galimberti, U. (1983) *Il corpo*, Milano: Feltrinelli.

—— (1984) *La terra senza il male*, Milano: Feltrinelli.

—— (1992) *Dizionario di psicologia*, Torino: UTET.

Gallant, C. (1978) *Blake and the Assimilation of Chaos*, Princeton: Princeton University Press.

Gandhi, M. K. (1958) *Antiche come le montagne*, Milano: Edizioni di Comunità, 1973.

Gardner, H. (1983) *Formae mentis. Saggio sulla pluralità dell'intelligenza*, Milano: Feltrinelli, 1987.

Gasca, G. (1993) 'Elementi per una teoria dei ruoli a partire dalla psicodramma', *Psicodramma Analitico*, 1, pp. 9–31, Torino: UPSEL.

Gasca, G. and Gasseau, M. (1991) *Lo psicodramma analitico*, Torino: Bollati Boringhieri.

Gergen, K. (1991) *The Saturated Self*, New York: Basic Books.

Gerra, G. and Frati, F. (2000) La ricerca sui disturbi psichiatrici nei pazienti tossicodipendenti ed alcolisti, in *Personalità/dipendenze*, vol. 6, Fascicolo I, pp. 73–87, Modena: Mucchi.

Gersie, A. (1996) *Dramatic Approaches to Brief Therapy*, London: Jessica Kingsley.

—— (1997) *Reflections on Therapeutic Storymaking*, London: Jessica Kingsley.

Giddens, A. (1991) *Modernity and Self-Identity*, Stanford: Stanford University Press.

Goffman, E. (1959) *La vita quotidiana come rappresentazione*, Bologna: Il Mulino, 1969.

—— (1961) *Asylums*, Torino: Edizioni di Comunità, 2001.

—— (1974) *Frame Analysis*, Roma: Armando, 2001.

Goleman, D. (1995) *L'intelligenza emotiva*, Milano: Rizzoli, 1996.

Gombrowicz, W. (1965) *Cosmo*, Milano: Feltrinelli, 1966.

Goodman, N. (1968) *I linguaggi dell'arte*, EST: Milano, 1998.

—— (1978) *Vedere e costruire il mondo*, Bari: Laterza, 1988.

Grainger. R. (1974) *The Language of Rite*, London: Darton, Longman & Todd.

—— (1990) *Drama and Healing*, London: Jessica Kingsley.

—— (1995) *The Glass of Heaven: The Faith of a Dramatherapist*, London: Jessica Kingsley.

—— (1999) *Researching the Arts Therapies*, London: Jessica Kingsley.

—— (2000) *Immaginazione e benessere*, in: 'Arte e Trasformazione'. Atti del convegno, Palermo: Coop. 'Il Canto di Los'.

Grainger, R. and Andersen-Warren, M. (2000) *Practical Approaches to Dramatherapy*, London: Jessica Kingsley.

Grainger, R. and Duggan, M. (1997) *Imagination, Identification and Catharsis in Theatre and Therapy*, London: Jessica Kingsley.

Grotowski, J. (1968) *Per un teatro povero*, Roma: Bulzoni, 1970.

Hesse, H. (1917) *Demian*, in Romanzi, Milano: Mondadori, 1977.

Hillman, J. (1983) *Le storie che curano*, Milano: Cortina, 1984.

—— (1996) *Il codice dell'anima*, Milano: Adelphi, 1997.

Hofmannsthal, H. von (1932) *Andrea o i ricongiunti*, Milano: Adelphi, 1970.

Huizinga, J. (1939) *Homo ludens*, Torino: Einaudi, 1973.

Huxley, A. (1932) *Il mondo nuovo*, Milano: Mondadori, 1933.

—— (1945) *La Filosofia Perenne*, Milano: Adelphi, 1995.

—— (1952) *I diavoli di Loudun*, Milano: Mondadori, 1960.

—— (1962) *L'isola*, Milano: Mondadori, 1963.

Jedlowski, P. (2000) *Storie comuni. La narrazione nella vita quotidiana*, Milano: Bruno Mondadori.

Jeffers, R. (1925) *La Bipenne e altre poesie*, Parma: Guanda, 1969.

Jenkyns, M. (1996) *The Play's the Thing*, London: Routledge.

Jennings, S. (1978) *Remedial Drama*, London: A. & C. Black.

—— (1988) 'Dramatherapy and groups', in S. Jennings (ed.) *Dramatherapy. Theory and Practice 1*, London: Routledge.

—— (1990) *Dramatherapy with Families, Groups and Individuals*, London: Jessica Kingsley.

—— (ed.) (1992) *Dramatherapy. Theory and Practice 2*, London: Routledge.

—— (1995a) *Theatre, Ritual and Transformation*, London: Routledge.

—— (ed.) (1995b) *Dramatherapy with Children and Adolescents*, London: Routledge.

—— (ed.) (1995c) *The Handbook of Dramatherapy*, London: Routledge.

—— (ed.) (1997) *Dramatherapy. Theory and Practice 3*, Routledge: London.

—— (1998) *Introduction to Dramatherapy*, London: Jessica Kingsley.

Jennings, S. and Minde, A. (1993) *Art Therapy and Dramatherapy. Masks of the Soul*, London: Jessica Kingsley.

Jervis, G. (1975) *Manuale critico di psichiatria*, Milano: Feltrinelli.

—— (1997) *La conquista dell'identità*, Milano: Feltrinelli.

Johnson, D. R., (1981) 'Drama therapy and the schizofrenic condition', in G. Schattner and R. Courtney *Drama in Therapy. Volume Two: Adults*, New York: Drama Book Specialists, pp. 47–66.

Johnstone, K. (1979) *Impro*, New York: Routledge.

—— (1999) *Impro for Storytellers*, New York: Routledge.

Jung, C. G. (1912/1952) *Simboli della trasformazione*, in *Opere*, vol. 5, Torino: Boringhieri, 1970.

—— (1921) *Tipi psicologici*, in *Opere*, vol. 6, Torino: Boringhieri, 1969.

—— (1928) *L'Io e l'inconscio*, in *Opere*, vol. 7, Torino: Boringhieri, 1983.

—— (1938–1940) *Psicologia e religione*, in *Opere*, vol. 11, Torino: Boringhieri, 1970.

—— (1950) *Sul rinascere*, in *Opere*, vol. 9, Torino: Boringhieri, 1980.

—— (1955/56) *Mysterium Coniunctionis*, in *Opere*, vol. 14, Torino: Boringhieri, 1989.

Kast, V. (1988) *Immaginazione attiva*, Como: RED, 1997.

Kelly, G. A. (1963) *A Theory of Personality*, New York: Norton.

Kerényi, K. (1963) *Gli dei e gli eroi della Grecia*, Milano: Il Saggiatore, 1963.

—— (1976) *Dioniso*, Milano: Adelphi, 1992.

Koestler, A. (1972) *Le radici del caso*, Roma: Astrolabio, 1972.

Kumiega, J. (1985) *Jerzy Grotowski*, Firenze: La Casa Usher, 1989.

La Cecla, F. (1997) *Il malinteso*, Bari: Laterza.

Lahad, M. (1992) 'Storymaking in assessment method for coping with stress: six-piece-story-making and BASICPh', in S. Jennings (ed.) *Dramatherapy. Theory and Practice 2*, London: Routledge, pp. 150–63.

—— (2000) *Creative Supervision*, London: Jessica Kingsley.

Laing, R. D. (1959) *L'io diviso*, Torino: Einaudi, 1969.

Landolfi, T. (1958) *Ottavio di Saint Vincent*, Milano: Rizzoli, 1979.

Landy, R. J. (1986) *Drammaterapia, concetti, teorie e pratica*, Roma: Edizioni Universitarie Romane, 1999.

—— (1993) *Persona and Performance*, London: Jessica Kingsley.

—— (1995) 'The dramatic world view: reflections on the roles taken and played by young children', in S. Jennings (ed.) *Dramatherapy with Children and Adolescents*, London: Routledge, pp. 7–27.

—— (1996) *The Double Life. Essays in Drama Therapy*, London: Jessica Kingsley.

Lazarus, R. S. (1982) 'Stress and coping as factors in health and illness', in J. Cohen *et al.* (eds) *Psychosocial Aspects of Cancer*, New York: Raven Press.

Leopardi, G. (1831) 'Canti', in *Tutte le opere*, vol. 3, Firenze: Sansoni, 1969.

Lewis, P. and Johnson, D. R. (2000) *Current Approaches in Drama Therapy*, Springfield, IL: C. C. Thomas.

Lorenz, K. (1983) *Il declino dell'uomo*, Milano: Mondadori, 1985.

McAdams, D. (1993) *The Stories We Live By*, NewYork: Guilford Press.

Marcelli, D. and Braconnier, A. (1983) *Psicopatologia dell'adolescenza*, Milano: Masson, 1985.

Marcuse, H. (1968) 'La liberazione dalla società opulenta', in D. Cooper (a cura di) *Dialettiche della liberazione*, Torino: Einaudi, 1969.

Maslow, A. (1962), *Verso una psicologia dell'essere*, Roma: Astrolabio, 1971.

Maturana, H. and Varela, F. (1980) *Autopoiesi e cognizione*, Venezia: Marsilio, 1985.

Mauss, M. (1950) *Teoria generale della magia*, Torino: Einaudi, 1965.

Mead, G. H. (1934) *Mente, sé e società*, Firenze: Giunti-Barbera, 1966.

Melucci, A. (a cura di) (1994) *Creatività: miti, discorsi, processi*, Milano: Feltrinelli.

Menegazzo, C. (1996) Lavorare con l'immaginario per ritrovare la soglia dell'umano, *Psicodramma Analitico* 5, pp. 45–56, Torino: UPSEL.

Mitchell, S. (ed.) (1996) *Dramatherapy: Clinical Studies*, London: Jessica Kingsley.

Morante, E. (1968) *Il mondo salvato dai ragazzini*, Torino: Einaudi.

Moreno, J. L. (1923) *Il teatro della spontaneità*, Firenze: Guaraldi, 1973.

—— (1946) *Manuale di psicodramma*, vol. I, Roma: Astrolabio, 1985.

—— (1959) *Gli spazi dello psicodramma*, Roma: Di Renzo, 1995.

—— (1969) *Manuale di psicodramma*, vol. II, Roma: Astrolabio, 1987.

Morin, E. (1986) *La conoscenza della conoscenza*, Milano: Feltrinelli, 1989.

Otto, R. (1917) *Il sacro*, Milano: Feltrinelli, 1984.

Pagnini, M. (1994) 'Introduzione', in William Blake, *Jerusalem*, Firenze: Giunti.

Paley, M. D. (1970) *Energy and Imagination. A Study of the Development of Blake's Thought*, Oxford: Oxford University Press.

Percival, M. O. (1937) *William Blake's Circle of Destiny*, reprinted by Kessinger Publishing Co., Montana, undated.

Perussia, F. (2000) *Storia del soggetto. La formazione mimetica della persona*, Torino: Bollati Boringhieri.

Pessoa, F. (1942) *Imminenza dell'ignoto*, Milano: Accademia, 1972.

Petrella, F. (1985) *La mente come teatro*, Torino: Centro Scientifico Torinese.

Pickering, K. (1997) *Drama Improvised*, Colwall: Garnet Miller.

Pieri, P. F. (1998) *Dizionario Junghiano*, Torino: Bollati Boringhieri.

Pitruzzella, S. (1995) 'Dall'animazione teatrale al teatro come terapia', *Artiterapie* 2, pp. 4–6.

—— (1998) 'Lo sguardo e la maschera', *Qu. Ar. Ter.* 1, pp. 6–10.

—— (2000) 'Drammaterapia', in C. Palazzi and A. Taverna *Arti Terapie. I fondamenti*, Torino: Tirrenia Stampatori.

—— (2002) 'States of grace. Transformative events in Dramatherapy', *Dramatherapy Journal* 24, 2, pp. 3–9, London: British Association of Dramatherapists.

Platone, *Fedro*, trad. di E. Martini, Milano: Sansoni, 1993.

Porter, R. (1987) *Storia sociale della follia*, Milano: Garzanti, 1991.

Pozzi, E. and Minoia V. (a cura di) (1999) *Di alcuni teatri della diversità*, Pesaro: Nuove Catarsi.

Raine, K. (1991) *Golgonooza, City of Imagination*, Hudson: Lindisfarne Press.

Ricoeur, P. (1990) *Sé come un altro*, Milano: Jaca Book, 1993.

—— (1992) *La persona*, Brescia: Morcelliana, 1997.

Rilke, R. M. (1900) *Le store del buon Dio*, Milano: Rizzoli, 1978.

—— (1923) *Elegie Duinesi*, Torino: Einaudi, 1978.

Rogers, C. R. (1961) *La terapia centrata sul cliente*, Firenze: Martinelli, 1970.

Ruggeri, V. (2001) *L'identità in psicologia e teatro*, Roma: Edizioni Scientifiche Magi.

Salas, J. (1993) *Improvising Real Life*, New Paltz: Tusitala, 1999.

Santagostino, P. (1987) 'Curarsi con le fiabe', *Riza Scienze* 17, Milano: Riza Edizioni.

Sarbin, T. and Allen, V. (1968) 'Role theory', in G. Lindzey and E. Aronson (eds) *The Handbook of Social Psychology*, 2nd ed, Reading: Addison-Wesley.

Sarbin, T. (ed.) (1986) *Narrative Psychology*, New York: Praeger.

Schattner, G. and Courtney, R. (1981) *Drama in Therapy. Volume Two: Adults*, New York: Drama Book Specialists.

Schechner, R. (1983) *La teoria della performance*, Roma: Bulzoni, 1984.

—— (1977/1993) *Magnitudini della performance*, Roma: Bulzoni, 1999.

Scheff, T. J. (1979) *Catharsis in Healing, Ritual and Drama*, Berkeley: University of California Press.

Schilder, P. (1935) *Immagine di sé e schema corporeo*, Milano: Franco Angeli, 1992.

Schotz, A. (1998) *Theatre Games and Beyond*, Colorado Springs: Meriwether.

Schutzenberger, A. A. (1970) *Le psicodramma*, Firenze: Martinelli, 1972.

Schwob, M. (1892) *Il re dalla maschera d'oro*, Bergamo: Moizzi.

Simmel, G. (1908–1920/21) *Filosofia dell'attore*, Pisa: ETS, 1998.

Slade, P. (1954) *Child Drama*, London: University of London Press.

Slade, P. (1968) *Experience of Spontaneity*, London: Longman.

Slade, P. (1995) *Child Play. Its Importance for Human Development*, London: Jessica Kingsley.

Spolin, V. (1963) *Improvisation for the Theater*, Evanston: Northwestern University Press.

—— (1986) *Theater Games for the Classroom*, Evanston: Northwestern University Press.

—— (1989) *Theater Game File*, Evanston: Northwestern University Press.

Stanislavskij, K. (1963) *Il lavoro dell'attore su se stesso*, Bari: Laterza, 1996.

Stein, E. (1917) *L'empatia*, Milano: Franco Angeli, 1985.

Stevenson, R.L. (1906) *A Child's Garden of Verses*, New York: Current Literature Publishing Co.

Tagore, R. (1903) *Sissu* (Canto d'infanzia), Parma: Guanda, 1979.

Tarkovskij, A. (1986) *Scolpire il tempo*, Milano: Ubulibri, 1988.

Taviani, F. (a cura di) (1975) *Il libro dell'Odin*, Milano: Feltrinelli.

Trombetta, C. (1989) *La creatività. Un'utopia contemporanea*, Milano: Bompiani.

Tselikas-Portmann, E. (1999) *Supervision and Dramatherapy*, London: Jessica Kingsley.

Turner,V. (1982) *Dal rito al teatro*, Bologna: Il Mulino, 1986.

—— (1986) *Antropologia della performance*, Bologna: Il Mulino, 1993.

Upaniṣad, a cura di C. della Casa, Torino: UTET, 1976.

Van Gennep, A. (1909) *I riti di passaggio*, Torino: Boringhieri, 1981.

Warren, B. (1981) *Drama Games*, North York: Captus Press.

Wiener, D. (1994) *Rehearsals for Growth*, New York: Norton.

—— (1999) *Beyond Talk Therapy*, Washington: American Psychological Association.

Wiesel, E. (1964) *Le porte della foresta*, Milano: Longanesi, 1989.

Wilshire, B. (1982) *Role-Playing and Identity. The Limits of Theatre as Metaphor*, Bloomington: Indiana University Press.

—— (1998) *Wild Hunger. The Primal Roots of Modern Addiction*, Lanham: Rowman & Littlefield.

Winnicott, D. W. (1971) *Gioco e realtà*, Roma: Armando, 1979.

Yalom, I. (1970) *Teoria e pratica della psicoterapia di gruppo*, Torino: Boringhieri, 1974.

Zapparoli, G. C. (1987) *La psicosi e il segreto*, Torino: Boringhieri.

Zoja, L. (1985) *Nascere non basta. Iniziazione e tossicodipendenza*, Milano: Cortina.

Dramatherapy on the internet

Applied and Interactive Theatre Guide: http://home.nyu.edu/~as245/AITG/

British Association for Dramatherapists: www.badth.co.uk/

Centro di Formazione nelle ArtiTerapie: www.artiterapie.it/

Dramatherapy in Greece and Cyprus: www.dramatherapy.gr

Dramatherapy Network (Sue Jennings website): www.dramatherapy.net/

National Association of Drama Therapists (USA): www.nadt.org

Index